Help!

I Can't Stop Eating

GETTING TO THE ROOT OF
YOUR OVEREATING

LANA ZINCONE

with Kim Cutulle

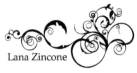

Copyright © 2013 Lana Zincone

ISBN—10: 1467923761
ISBN—13: 9781467923767

Cover Design: CreateSpace
Cover Photograph & Lana Zincone Photograph: Ema Suvajac
Kim Cutulle Photograph: Paula Cutulle

DEDICATION

....

Lana Zincone

It has been said that in life, we never stop learning. I also believe that in life, we never stop growing emotionally. This book is lovingly dedicated to my daughter, Tara, my sons, Aaron and Nolan, and those of us who choose to continue a lifelong journey along the path of learning and growing.

Kim Cutulle

I dedicate this book to my daughters, Sydney and Maya, whose beauty, innocence, and trust in life, and all the amazing things it has to offer, have been my inspiration and motivation – and to my husband, Mario, not only for all his patience with the many long hours and late nights spent alone, but also for his unwavering support in this project.

Contents

Acknowledgments

To Kim Cutulle, what can I say...without you, your devoted support and constant encouragement in this project, as well as the long hours and late nights spent working, not to mention your optimism and endless patience, there would be no book.

Susan Jamieson, President and CEO, Food Diva Inc., has been a great source of encouragement and support. I appreciate the many hours spent, over coffee, imparting your insight and vision while sharing creative marketing ideas and strategies for this book. Your professionalism and desire to make a difference are a standout.

Rob Nickel, Professional Speaker and Author of *Staying Safe in a Wired World,* thank you for taking time out of your busy schedule to advise and provide me with valuable information on all matters promotional. Your lighthearted, easy approach and humour have given me the confidence to move forward and speak in public.

Audrey Wilson, President and CEO, Gemini Modelling Agency, thank you for your continued support and help in promoting this book.

Tara Akuna and Joyce Harry, thank you for your encouragement and for tolerating the endless emails asking you to once again read over the chapters to give your comments, opinions, and valuable feedback.

Thanks to my husband, Mike Williams, for his expertise in the world of finance regarding publication and promotion.

Our families, for their love, support, and understanding and for their patience in having to put up with our obsession about this book and the endless phone calls back and forth.

INTRODUCTION

....

Why I Didn't Write This Book 25 Years Ago

Once we work on the underlying cause of our problem,
we will be able to let go of the weight
we have been holding on to.

Recently I was asked why it took me 25 years before I decided to write this book. I was surrounded by many others who, like me, were also struggling with weight problems of their own. The difference was that I recognized my overeating was not just about food; I knew it went much deeper than that. It was about what was driving me to overeat, the underlying reasons for the persistent binges that had become my frequent companion.

Throughout my early teens and mid-twenties, I had such a difficult time losing weight and keeping it off. I practically starved myself just to notice a difference. I was so intensely focused on what I was eating or what I was going to eat and consequently spent an inordinate amount of time counting calories, weighing myself, and perusing the latest diet. As a result, I was unable to concentrate on little else.

My personal library consisted of the latest diet books, but the irony of it was that after all this time, I found myself still fighting with my weight, now even heavier than before. I concluded that I had a slow metabolism or a thyroid problem. The unfortunate truth was that I had neither.

I always felt as though I were suffering inside, a kind of suffering no one understood. Food had such a hold over me, and as much as I was completely drawn to it, I also feared the power it held, yet I was not content to assign myself to the fact that this would be a lifetime struggle.

With fierce determination I began my search for the answer, and with the help of a friend, developed a Method of finding the root of my problem. Once I had worked out the reasons why I was so dependent on food, my problem very quickly resolved itself. I no longer experienced the continual internal struggle that was so familiar to me. Within a short period of time I began to lose weight and my overeating ended.

I also discovered that when we have negative experiences, past or present, one of our body's natural defenses is to gain weight and hold on to it as a form of self-preservation. This is one of the many defense mechanisms we subconsciously employ when faced with emotional pain. I realized this was my way of protecting myself physically, as well as emotionally, and looking back over past experiences, I could see how I had used my weight as a protective barrier. My belief is that once we work on the underlying cause of our struggle with food, we will then be able to let go of the weight we have been holding on to.

Twenty-five years ago the connection had yet to be made in finding the underlying reasons why we crave and overeat; however, as the years passed, I watched others not only fail to lose the excess weight but, in the process, gain more. Simply put, after all these years they still struggle.

Even with a healthy lifestyle and proper nutrition at the forefront of today's thinking, we still manage to succumb to the lure of the latest diet's promise to melt off x number of pounds in just two short weeks. Like everything else, things evolve and progress, and even though today there is a profusion of seemingly limitless information about this connection, there still does not appear to be a concrete, non-evasive method to eradicate it altogether. Furthermore, the number of people who struggle with this problem continues to grow exponentially.

This book is unique in that it does not dictate diet or exercise plans but addresses the underlying reasons why we are in this cycle of dieting and overeating. This Method will not only provide you with the insight and tools needed to find the root of your problem, but will also guide you step by step how to overcome it yourself. It will show you an easier, less painful way to stop this behaviour.

You will become more relaxed around food and naturally stop when you feel you've had enough. With the absence of craving and overeating, your weight will no longer fluctuate because you won't feel the urge to eat out of control. Your main focus will not be on dieting, and for perhaps the first time in a long time, you will be able to turn your attention to other areas of your life that have been neglected. Everything will change. Your outlook on life will change. Future prospects will hold an excitement that was previously only reserved for the first fleeting moments of a binge. You will feel more powerful and find it easier to embrace new challenges in life. Most importantly, this change will leave you feeling more in control, more positive, more at ease, and infinitely more at peace.

As a result of people wanting to know how I managed to keep the weight off all these years, I was motivated to put pen to paper and write this book in the hope of sharing it with those who, like myself, have struggled and suffered far too long.

In writing this book, it is my intention to further change the relationship you have with food, as well as your perception about weight loss. Overcoming your struggle is possible, and I believe that if I can teach my Method through the sharing of my own personal experience, then perhaps I can help put an end to this problem.

1

STILL SEARCHING FOR THAT MAGIC PILL

....

Why Dieting Doesn't Work

*Our struggle with food can fool us into thinking
we don't have a problem,
which is why we continue to believe
the newest regimen will finally be the one.*

Statistics show obesity continues to be on the rise. Why is this most apparent when not only have we been educated about the absolute importance of a healthy lifestyle, but also now more than ever enjoy this abundance of information critical to improving and extending our lives at the mere touch of a button? Could it perhaps be the continual cycle of dieting and overeating? For years, experts have attempted to answer these questions, among others.

These experts believe that the way to freedom from this destructive behaviour is through changing our relationship with food, thereby changing the way we eat. They refer to this as a lifestyle change. And when the body and mind become disciplined in this lifestyle change, then it should be permanent. Sadly, this assumption has many times been proven incorrect. Numerous studies contradict this as evidence shows that when we reintroduce these foods back into our lives, for many it only reawakens our taste buds, our sleeping giant, generating the overeating that follows and resulting in this cycle once again.

The 1960's ushered in a new decade that changed the face of not only our political landscape and standard of living, but also how we as women defined ourselves and what role we chose to play in society.

Women were now independent, many trading their aprons for suits, seeking to climb the corporate ladder rather than remain in the typist pool or be secretary to the boss. Beauty underwent radical changes, from the voluptuous ultrafeminine sex symbols of the 1950's to the bra-burning, freethinking women of the 1960's. The ideal woman was now typified by an extremely thin Twiggy, one of the top models of the day, and we seem after all these years unable to break free of this standard. This body type represents a very small percentage of the population, leaving the rest struggling to achieve this unrealistic and unattainable goal. It further sends the message when a variety of current magazines routinely display pictures of exceedingly thin celebrities and the extremes they are willing to go through in order to achieve this look. Their battle with weight has become fodder for intense public scrutiny, sending a clear message that being overweight is unacceptable, period.

I strongly believe that the process of dieting is in part responsible for the overeating problems and resultant obesity that are rampant in our society. When we diet, we restrict ourselves from the very foods we crave. And when we restrict ourselves, we begin to think about these foods and ultimately obsess about them. The cravings may become so intensified that they permeate our every thought and our very being. If we were told not to think of a chocolate fudge cake, it's very unlikely that we could think of little else, our mouths watering as we imagine the taste and texture of it. This is a fine example of the power of suggestion.

How often has someone on a diet sat down to enjoy a favourite TV show, possibly to divert her thoughts away from food, and found herself flooded with commercial after commercial hawking all the forbidden foods? At this point, many become overwhelmed with cravings, seeking refuge in whatever happens to be in the kitchen. When we're told what we can't have, we automatically want it because it's human nature, and dieting is just that. It's dictating that we can't eat the very things we enjoy.

When we diet, we deprive ourselves, causing our metabolism to slow down in an attempt to conserve fat and energy, thus prolonging the process of losing weight. This occurs because our body is desperately holding on to what it perceives as its last meal. Historically, this is our genetic response because food was not readily available on a daily basis, leaving us for extended periods without eating. When we did eat, we would consume as much as we possibly could in preparation for the next fast. As a result, we may find ourselves hitting a plateau. In frustration, we begin to eat less and exercise more. Feeling that the whole process is futile, we succumb to our cravings, gaining the weight back even quicker and easier than before.

Restricting our intake will also deplete our energy, leaving us feeling weak and lethargic. This physical state is difficult to sustain, and in order to re-energize, we turn to food, but more often than not once we start, we're unable to stop. This is our body's way of overcompensating to make up for lost calories throughout this period.

We may question the merit of a healthy, balanced diet, one that isn't drastic. This might work fine for some, but it is still a diet, and as such I see it as a restriction that will perpetuate cravings.

When we begin to incorporate some of these foods back into our diet, this may be all that is needed to trigger old habits. One small dessert may soon become two, until eventually we find that our clothes begin to feel tighter, and before we know it, we've gained back the weight and possibly even more. And so the destructive cycle begins once again.

When we are in the midst of a craving, we are unable to think rationally and therefore have a difficult time identifying our thoughts or feelings. As a result we find ourselves turning to food without even realizing it. Therein lies the danger. This hunger is much different from the normal hunger we experience as there seems to be no limit to what we can consume. When we are driven by this hunger, food does not fill us because, regardless of what we eat, we never truly feel satisfied.

There were days when I could literally eat from morning until night, yet I never felt satisfied. I only craved more. Once I finished the pastries and the chocolate bars, I was then looking for the chips, and after the chips it was ice cream. Then and only then, when there was nothing left to consume, would I feel completely and utterly stuffed. I was left feeling physically ill, exhausted, and ashamed that I once again succumbed to this gluttony. No matter how much we consume, we are always left with a feeling of indescribable emptiness.

But I Don't Have a Problem

Your struggle with food can in many ways be a problem in disguise. It can fool you into thinking you don't have a problem, which is why so many of us, after years of dieting and exercise programs, continue to believe the newest regimen will finally be the one that will be successful. There are those days when our cravings and appetites are insatiable, yet there are other days where we have no problem controlling what and how much we eat. This in itself becomes deceptive because our eating patterns are not always consistent.

For some women, our appetites increase substantially with the onset of menses, and often these cravings are for high-fat, sugary, starchy foods. We eat and eat for a week straight, perpetuating a one-to-two week cycle of craving and overeating, only to then starve ourselves in an attempt to get back on track.

Some of us believe if we just find the right diet our problem will be gone for good. Or we don't have a problem dieting and getting the weight off, it's just a matter of keeping it off. For many of us, our days begin feeling normal and in control, but by the time night falls, we succumb to our usual pattern of overeating. The next morning, we wake up believing we're fine because we are feeling strong, it's a new day, and we convince ourselves that this time we will be in control. But somehow it never seems to happen, and once the evening hours approach, the temptation strikes again without warning.

I listen to many women complain about their weight and how they are unable to get it off and keep it off. They admit to having a poor body image and would never entertain the thought of stepping into a bathing suit, let alone going to the beach. Some are unable to relax and enjoy intimacy because they are so self-conscious of their appearance and how they perceive themselves. As one woman said, "When I get out of bed, I always make sure the lights are dim, and I never let my husband see me without any clothes on. God forbid, he would ever touch me again!" After many years and many conversations, it still pains me to hear these unchanging comments, having experienced the same low self-esteem that accompanied my perception of feeling unattractive and overweight.

Looking back, I remember just how much this interfered with my life and the amount of energy that was spent on it. It robbed me of a great deal of my youth when it should have been a more carefree time. Now 25 years later, at the age of 54, I know that many of these women have gone through the same experience most of their lives, for some, 30 to 40 years. This frustrates me because I overcame this problem 25 years ago, and I want people to understand that this no longer needs to be the focus of their lives. It can be overcome with the right understanding and methodology.

Unfortunately, when I talk to these women about how to overcome their struggle, I feel they're in denial. They say things such as, "I'm okay, my only problem is that I eat in the evening. If I just kept myself busy at night, I'd be alright." "I don't have a problem getting the weight off, it's just keeping it off." "If I just stuck to an exercise program, I'd be okay." "It's hormonal." "I just don't have the time right now."

We never manage to reach our ideal weight, and life becomes a seemingly endless roller-coaster ride of weight gain and weight loss, leaving us feeling emotionally and physically exhausted. Strangely, not unlike the gambler who holds out for that one big win, we continue to remain fooled, holding on to the hope that the next diet will be our big win, ultimately transforming our lives.

Over the last 30 years, I have listened to excuses of every description, and these are the very excuses that prevent people from dealing with the real issues of why they're overeating in the first place. If there were an opportunity to get down to their ideal weight without the restrictions diets offer, hands down, they would jump at the chance. However, it appears some people live their lives justifying their behaviour by inadvertently focusing on the wrong things. In looking beyond the diet, they may come to the realization that their problem is connected to something other than food. The focus needs to be on why they're overeating and how to resolve it.

A colleague, married for over 20 years, still finds it hard to believe that some members of his wife's family have been on a perpetual diet since they first met. And he adds, "They look the same now as they did when I first met them, with the exception of a few more pounds." It's ironic that even after all this time, these same people are still dieting, still searching for that magic pill to totally transform their bodies. What they fail to realize is they need to look beyond food as this will not be solved by repeated unsuccessful attempts at dieting.

Is There a Quick Fix?
Many are caught up with what I refer to as the "quick fix" method of losing weight such as the low-carb

diet, the low-fat diet, the high-protein diet, and the list virtually goes on and on. Not to mention cosmetic surgeries and procedures, mainly liposuction, tummy tucks, and gastric bypass surgery. Our society is impatient in that we want it yesterday and furthermore have become accustomed as such. So many of us have been fooled by these methods, holding on to the false hope that one of them will actually work and render us permanently thin.

There is no such thing as a quick fix when it comes to successful weight loss. In my experience and that of countless others, quick fix methods are not the quick way at all; they're often the long road to failure. They are only temporary at best, and generally people find they never get down to their ideal weight with them. I have witnessed many others over the years attempt numerous weight loss methods, and today, 25 years later, these same people are still tempted and persuaded by them. This isn't simply a love of food; it's not about food at all. It's about why we are craving and overeating in the first place. In order to overcome this, we need to realize that the real quick fix is to find the root cause of our problem and resolve it there, as this will result in permanent change.

Many of us fail to see that our overeating can stem from an underlying source. We may feel as though we are just enjoying our food, but have you noticed most times when you are overeating it occurs when you're not hungry? How then does this happen? When we hold on to issues from our past that for whatever reason have not been dealt with – times when, during our youth, we were told we were not good enough, smart enough, or attractive enough – we would, as a result, take on these beliefs as our own. We may feel because these experiences happened in the past they have been long forgotten, no longer affecting us. But nothing could be further from the truth. If these past experiences remain unresolved, they will then re-emerge in the form of an uncomfortable feeling or emotion, one we neither recognize nor know what to do with. And this disconcerting emotion will inevitably elicit cravings within us, driving us to search for an outlet such as food, drugs, or alcohol in order to fill them. If these outlets manage to give us relief, they will do so temporarily, in the end, serving only to make things worse. And the emotion that has been appeased or suppressed with food will return once again.

Therapists now understand there is a reason behind the driving force that causes us to crave and succumb to those cravings by eating to excess. For some it has taken many years of weekly sessions under the guidance of a trained professional to find the reason for this, yet others learn to live with it, managing so they can function in their lives. And many of these people continue to suffer each day not only struggling with their cravings, but also with the nagging and uncomfortable thought that there has to be a reason why they are behaving this way and what they can do to stop it.

After speaking to many people who, in the midst of their own struggle, asked me how I overcame mine, my response was that I accomplished this without dieting. It was ineffective because by restricting myself, I unknowingly perpetuated the cycle of dieting and overeating. I not only gained back the weight I had lost, but with each new diet managed to gain more. In short, it made things worse. And because restricting myself caused undue suffering, this was a feeling I no longer wanted to experience. Realizing that dieting was detrimental and soul-destroying, I had to find another solution, a different approach, because there was a reason why I couldn't control these cravings. I just had to find it and eventually did, using a Method I developed to locate the root of my problem.

Every evening before going to sleep, I made it a priority to visualize, which is a gentle approach and one of the main components of the Method. I found, with practice, my cravings and overeating began to subside, eventually becoming non-existent. Food ceased to be a daily struggle because for the first time in a long time I felt in control of my life.

So many years had been wasted fighting this battle, and, looking back, had I not persevered, I would have, in all likelihood, spent many more years or quite possibly my entire lifetime searching for that magic pill, that elusive answer. And I became hopeful in the knowledge that if my Method proved to be successful for me, then surely it would be successful for others.

2

BREAKING FREE FROM THE STRANGLEHOLD OUR DIET HAS OVER US

....

Struggling & Irrational Thinking

In life, when faced with difficulty,
we tend to focus on the problem itself
rather than finding the source, the root cause —
and so it is with our struggle.

When we diet, temptation becomes more apparent. Food we normally wouldn't think about is now our main focus, enticing us. The yo-yo dieting begins and we find ourselves in the midst of frustration, fighting to keep the weight off. We resort to drastic measures spending an inordinate amount of time starving ourselves and beating our bodies back into shape with excessive exercise.

We behave this way because we are constantly bombarded with a parade of endless advertisements and magazine articles, reams of diet books, and the influence of the media that lead us to believe the only way to gain control of our weight is through dieting. As a result, we end up focusing on the wrong aspect of the problem.

Emotionally, we go through an irrational thought process where we feel diets are the culprit. We accusingly point the finger at them, believing they're the reason for our pain and suffering. And if we're not blaming the diets, we're blaming the people who developed them. We question why they can't create a diet that will allow us to eat what we love and still lose weight without all the restrictions.

Traditionally, most occasions centre around food. "The breaking of the bread" brings people together, as evident in many cultures. And when we reflect on these occasions, food has always been the focus. In retrospect, people often recall an event by the food that was served. Unfortunately, we dread the thought of attending these social events because we feel we're no longer able to enjoy them. We worry about spending the evening grazing at the hors d'oeuvre table, only to wake up the next morning staring with contempt at our bathroom scales. And we're afraid that once we start we'll never stop. Then there are those events where we just can't seem to help ourselves from completely overdoing it, despite the fear our true identity will be revealed, leaving us at the wrath of others for sniffing around their plates after cleaning off ours.

I remember agonizing over whether or not to attend birthday parties. For me, they were torture because I knew it was proper etiquette and ladylike to accept only one piece of cake. I wondered how anyone could offer me just one piece, knowing it would never be enough. Imagine agonizing over attending social events, realizing your entire evening would be spent struggling with this internal dialogue.

Weight loss books state that in order to achieve our desired weight and remain there, we must make a permanent lifestyle change. This, however, can be misinterpreted in many ways, some irrational, leaving us to believe we'll never be able to enjoy the food we love, and constantly fighting the temptation to eat because the urge will always be there, lurking in the background.

When we control our urges we feel suppressed, as though we're locked up inside. This creates an internal struggle because we have an incredible desire to break free from the stranglehold our diet has over us. But we are unable to do so because we're desperately trying to lose weight. Over time, this results in feelings of deprivation and unhappiness, feelings that regrettably can only be appeased with food.

This cycle of craving and overeating continues, leaving our health compromised, ultimately carrying even more weight on our already bulging frames, not to mention the feelings of anger, remorse, and hopelessness that follow in its wake. The thought of not being able to enjoy the food we love can feel as though we've lost a best friend. We eventually reach the point where we become angry and rebel by eating the very things we can't have, only to find ourselves gaining back the weight we had previously lost.

In absolute frustration and nearing the end of our rope, we allow ourselves to be led down the garden path to try one more diet, which turns out to be just as restricting and unyielding as the previous one, ultimately leading us straight into the arms of yet another binge. Not unlike a mouse on a perpetual treadmill, we do this because this is what we've always done, so the cycle continues...unfortunately for some, for a lifetime.

The promise of yet another highly acclaimed diet was often too great for me to ignore, and I would therefore decide to try once again. In the beginning, I felt excited and energized, thinking it would be a new way of living for me as I was going to eat healthier, think healthier, and ultimately look healthier. I was to become this new person, just as the latest diet book proclaimed.

I would begin cleaning out my fridge and cupboards, planning my new meals, and buying all the required food. Mornings were encouraging, but as night approached, those old, nagging feelings crept up and I found myself becoming restless. Nothing seemed to take away that unsettling feeling. I tried watching TV, going for a walk, and reading a magazine, but found it difficult to concentrate. I tried re-reading some of the chapters in my new diet book for motivation and support while nibbling on the recommended snacks. However, when I managed to eat a week's worth in just under an hour, I knew I was headed for real trouble. I could feel those same familiar, tormenting feelings returning with a vengeance. And as I ate the chocolates, the cake, and the ice cream in the convenience store parking lot, that pressing, restless feeling would slowly dissolve, leaving me in a sea of remorse, guilt, and empty containers.

Regardless of how hard or how long we battle with this, we need to understand our struggle with food is in part emotional; therefore, it is essential to get to the root of why we are overeating, and in doing so, this will give us the strength and confidence in knowing we can resolve it.

This Method helped me overcome the cravings and overeating that up to this point had all but dominated my life. The cravings began to subside and, with it, the urgency to be ever watchful, ever vigilant.

The Method I have formulated is simple and straightforward, and once learned, you will be confident that you have a workable approach to overcome your struggle. As you experience a new sense of control, a subtle but amazing change will occur, and, with it, a feeling of all things possible.

3

FOR THE LAST TIME

....

My Personal Battle With Food

As humans, we have that innate ability
to fight the good fight—
even when we feel we haven't the strength.

I was raised in a household where food was the main focus. I remember eagerly looking forward to that one day each week when my father would arrive home with the long-awaited groceries, and I knew if I wasn't home at just the right time to welcome them into the kitchen, I would risk missing out on all the "good stuff." Coming from a large family, food never lasted very long because anything that entered our house was instantly consumed out of fear that someone else would get to it first.

It was common, given these circumstances, for me to feel that I never got enough. Of course we did get dessert once a week, and when it came we were like vultures diving in until it was all finished. All those open mouths eagerly devoured it in one fell swoop. The idea being, you made damn sure to eat as much as you possibly could because a second helping would be non-existent. This was survival, and it became my goal to figure out how I could get my share, and shamelessly sometimes more if I was crafty enough.

Looking at nature versus nurture, I believe my preoccupation with food stemmed from a combination of both. This was something passed down from my parents and their parents before them. Especially those that lived, suffered and were deprived throughout the Depression and the World Wars. My parents and I were raised in the "finish everything on your plate" era, which was more often than not accompanied with the guilt-provoking lecture about all the starving children in the world.

Losing my father at the age of 11 triggered an inherent dependency on food, in turn creating the overeating and subsequent problems that ensued. Whatever fears and uncertainties I sustained when hit with this unbearable tragedy became that much more pronounced. And, as a result, from this age forward, food became my security blanket, my comfort zone, my safe place, and my feel-good drug. I just wasn't happy unless I was eating. In the midst of my topsy-turvy world, in the midst of all the upheaval, food quite literally became my everything.

As time progressed, my appetite for sweets became so insatiable that you could never just offer me one piece of cake or a cookie because this would set me off on a tangent. At birthday parties, it was not uncommon to find me sneaking around cleaning the cake off everyone's plates. I don't think there was an event or emotion where I didn't overeat. When there was a celebration, I overate. When I was bored, I overate.

When I watched TV, I overate. When I was frustrated, I overate. I literally associated everything with food.

Over the years this struggle permeated my subconscious to the point where many of my dreams consisted of eating. They were so intense and real that the next morning I literally felt sick and full as though it had actually happened.

It wasn't difficult to eat three or four donuts at one sitting. My friends could not believe the amount I was capable of consuming at one time, as they were able to satisfy themselves with just one. If they only knew the extent of it, I could have easily eaten more and this wasn't even a serious binge.

I made it appear as a joke to cover up the fact that I was really out of control and not feeling very good about myself. My friends were convinced of this as they took a picture of me in my Donut Queen T-shirt, laughingly accepting six presumably full donut boxes. The joke amongst us was that one day I would open my own donut shop with my revolving head on the roof. I would laugh along with them and didn't get angry or upset as I knew it was all in fun. Neither they nor I had any idea how deep this problem went or where it was going.

Later on when it became apparent that I was struggling with my weight, I often felt people downplayed my suffering, telling me I didn't have a problem. They weren't a witness to the overeating and saw me only occasionally splurge on something I was enjoying immensely. They would look at me in comparison to their own weight, stating they had the problem, not me. In their opinion, my excess of 35 pounds was really nothing much to worry about. Ironically, my weight eventually went from being the biggest part of the picture to taking a back seat to the emotional turmoil I was going through.

Then there were others who felt they were an authority on the subject of my roller-coaster weight. They would give me offhand advice such as "Just exercise and you won't have a problem." I tried various forms of exercise, settling on bodybuilding, hoping I would look like those muscular women with thin hips and wide shoulders. Unfortunately it didn't work because in order to see muscle tone, I needed to lose the body fat. I also heard "Push yourself away from the table and don't eat. Fight it." This worked only for a short while because I felt so deprived, and with this constant internal battle I just could not stop thinking about food. Another comment was "You just need to find a diet that you like and stick to it. Once you've eaten this way for a while, you'll eventually stop craving the other stuff and you'll be okay." You've got to be kidding, stop eating cake and chocolate, not in this lifetime. Although when people said these things, I held on to the hope that they were right because just maybe they knew something I didn't.

All this advice eventually made me feel even more frustrated and helpless. Nothing worked. I would think, "It's easy for you to give me advice when you don't have this problem. Try living a few weeks in my skin and see how you feel." I came to the realization that people often undermined my problem because of their inability to understand my experience.

I never really perceived I had a volatile relationship with food until my teen years. I was so used to the way I ate that in some strange way I believed it to be normal. The importance of being thin was never more apparent. My girlfriend and I became obsessed with wanting to look like those models whose perfect faces and bodies accosted us from the pages of every fashion magazine. Little did we realize these pictures were the result not only of the many hours of preparation on the part of the makeup artists and the photographers' artistic talent in airbrushing, but also of the models who made a career out of starving themselves to achieve this look. As a result, we decided that in order to look as perfect as they did, we would have to put ourselves on a strict diet. The irony was, at the time, we were both relatively thin. But as far as we were concerned, not thin enough.

The night before our diet was spent eating large amounts of candy, ice cream, cake, and whatever else happened to appear in our line of vision. We convinced ourselves it was okay, as we reasoned it would be a very long time before we could enjoy these foods again. We made an event of it, our own private food party. You name it, we ate it, and as much as we possibly could. It not only stretched our stomachs, enabling us to eat that much more, but also kept us on a perpetual sugar high, craving and craving.

The next day, unable to hold back, found us once again breaking the diet and ravenously eating everything that crossed our path. Between mouthfuls we consoled each other, forgiving ourselves the transgression, then convincing ourselves tomorrow was going to be different. In the aftermath, sitting there bloated, stuffed, and surveying the damage, we once again swore a solemn oath that this time we really meant business. This was it. This newfound strength would transform our thoughts, leaving us with a reformed attitude. We would reign triumphant over this demon food, becoming thin and free, looking great, and feeling great.

However, sadly we were mistaken once again. The new diet of the day soon ended in a binge along with many more to follow. The more we ate, the more we craved, and the more we craved, the more we ate. Now there was even more weight to lose. The pressure to get it off escalated, and our diet became that much more strict and regimented. Consequently, it was even more difficult to abstain from what we craved. This destructive cycle marked the beginning of a tumultuous 14-year relationship with food. This unhealthy relationship made me miserable and depressed because it had such a hold over me, and I felt it held me back from accomplishing my dreams and goals. It prevented me from living, from being present, and from enjoying what life had to offer.

I also became disenchanted with all the hype surrounding exercise and how great it was supposed to make me look and feel. However, despite feeling this way, there were those times I was motivated just long enough to try one form or another. I did have some successful days sticking to a diet and exercise program, but as soon as the diet stopped, so, too, would the exercise.

I was never at peace with how I looked because my weight was always inconsistent and, as a result, so too were my emotions. The many times I gained weight I felt bloated and unhealthy, and this was the image I would outwardly project. I was fat and then thin, liking myself, then hating myself. This went on for years and when I achieved a weight where I was happy, it never lasted long. I lived in the very real fear I would regain it and hate myself all over again. And I always managed to live up to that fear.

In my desperate attempt to lose weight I began taking enemas and laxatives in order to flatten my stomach. I did this once, sometimes twice a day, and developed severe gastrointestinal problems. I also resorted to diet pills and Benzedrine, commonly known as "bennies." They gave me a feeling of excitement. My heart would beat faster, I could breathe deeper and had lots of drive and energy. I felt I was able to conquer anything I set my mind to. I would completely lose my appetite, which for me was a miracle in itself; however, as soon as the pills wore off, I made up for it by eating everything in sight.

In no time, I began to notice that the more I used these diet pills the less potent they became. I even noticed I was regaining my appetite while on them. Eventually I stopped taking them because I lost interest in something that proved ineffective. It didn't take long for me to find another quick fix that held the false promise of a fast and permanent solution.

In my search for ways to control myself I decided to consume my meals by chewing and then spitting them out. This way, I could enjoy my food yet not absorb the calories. I had heard this method was gaining popularity, not only with the international set but also with women of all ages and socioeconomic backgrounds. Unfortunately, this didn't work because once I started, the food tasted so good I could not help but swallow it.

Then out of complete desperation, I tried sticking my fingers down my throat to induce vomiting, but, fortunately for me, regardless of how hard I tried, I just could not purge. Purging would have afforded me the luxury of eating whatever I wanted while remaining thin; however, it would have also paved the way for the debilitating disorder, Bulimia. I was fully aware of the painful psychological damage and physical havoc incurred by those unfortunate enough to fall victim to this. I strongly believe to this day that had I been successful at purging, I would have avoided looking within and would have continued to run from my fears and ultimately myself.

I often wondered what kind of demon these cravings that possessed me were all about. When I gave into these powerful cravings, they would ultimately reward me by returning with more frequency and strength. In observing others, I knew I was not the same as they were. There was something different about me, about my eating habits, because I could feel this relentless driving force constantly pulling me toward the lure of food.

I felt other people regarded food as something to be enjoyed, even when they indulged, but that its main purpose was for sustenance. Food satiated them when they were hungry and once satisfied, they were effortlessly able to move on to other interests in life. My attention, however, focused solely on what I could eat today, and the next day, and the day after that. Planned evenings eating in front of the TV with my favourite foods occupied a great deal of my time and energy.

Often I would say, "I know I should stop eating but it's too late now. I'll start fresh tomorrow." Even though part of me loved these foods, another part hated the pain they brought. There was still yet another part of me that wanted to be able to enjoy them and stop at just one. It was at this point I realized the only thing that would stop this behaviour was not dieting but getting to the root of my problem. The question was how. Food, as much as I adored it, possessed a power over me I equally feared.

On the advice of a friend, I decided to attend a support group for people who struggled with overeating. Their primary goal was to learn how to abstain from what they referred to as compulsive overeating. It was a safe place where people could talk about what they were going through, the cravings, the binges, and falling off the wagon without fear of being judged.

I began to attend these weekly sessions and for a time felt I had come to the right place, that for sure this time I would be able to receive help and finally be normal. They held the belief that there are those who have an addiction to food and that this addiction was a disease that was incurable, something we would have to live with the rest of our lives. They felt that in order to control this disease, we would have to abstain from the foods that triggered binges, which in itself proved difficult because for me it wasn't always a specific type of food that set me off and running. Looking back, I realize food alone had the ability to trigger binges.

I wondered how I could possibly abstain from the very foods I loved, food from my childhood that I associated with celebrations, food that made me feel safe when there was no one or nothing else to turn to. This I was to do for the rest of my life? This then felt like another life sentence imposed upon me.

I often asked myself how and when I got this disease the support group referred to. How did this happen? I didn't recall having this as a young child, and I wasn't born with it, that much I knew. So where did it come from? As a child I enjoyed eating candy and desserts as most children do, but I also knew when I had had enough. I didn't remember constantly thinking about food, dreaming about it, or eating this way as a young child. So why then did I have to suffer from this incurable disease for the rest of my life?

It wasn't long before I realized I just could neither accept their theory nor share their belief. There had to be another way for me to overcome this, not just be content to live in its shadow. I wanted to turn back time and become who I once was – Normal. Consequently, I walked away from this support group and was again back on the road in search of a better answer, hopefully one with a permanent solution. I never gave up hope that I would find one, and I think that hope kept me searching.

While looking for the elusive answer, a close friend shared her belief about the origin of my problem. She was able to help me realize and somehow trust that many of my issues were connected to my father.

My father, whom I adored despite his domineering personality, also possessed a temper, which I equally feared. I had a strong desire to make him happy, fix what was wrong, and smooth things out. But it never worked. Regardless of what I did or how hard I tried, he would always find something to complain about.

I even did things that compromised my own happiness. My father often complained that we never took care of our toys and how they always ended up in pieces. One Christmas, I took some of my board games and put them unopened, high on my closet shelf. They lay untouched for three months. I remember one winter afternoon, when I was playing with my brothers and sister, my father came into my room to talk to us. I told him I had a surprise for him as I opened the closet door and pointed to the top shelf. When I showed him how well I was taking care of my board games, keeping them brand-new, there was no response. He just stood there, saying nothing. When I looked at him, I saw a far-off, distant gaze. It seemed as though he had his mind on something else. I couldn't understand why, after all his complaining about our toys, he would not be proud of me. I was so sure if I showed him how well I took care of them, keeping them brand-new, then surely it would make him happy. It didn't.

Even though it saddened and hurt me at this young and impressionable age, I somehow convinced myself it was okay, it was just the way he was. His lack of interest was appropriate, for him. Later I was to see how, as a result of my acceptance of his behaviour, this lack of interest would be further tolerated in future relationships. What I also couldn't have understood was how difficult an adjustment it was for him to marry late in life and then have five children barely a year apart. He had gone from quiet bachelorhood to a very busy and loud existence in just a few short years. Somehow I don't think it was his original plan.

Looking back, this demonstrates the depth of a child's unconditional love for a parent. For me to sacrifice playing with my new toys to please my father was an indication of how much I wanted and needed his approval. I looked up to my father and wanted to be just like him. I needed his love and affection but received it only on his terms. My father was not an overly demonstrative man, but I believe he was more than capable of expressing these feelings because of his ability to give of himself freely when he chose. This inconsistent pattern of having love and affection given to me, then withheld, often and without provocation, featured prominently in many relationships of my young adulthood.

I sometimes felt my parents were absentee parents. They seemed much too preoccupied and distracted a great deal of the time to really pay attention. I had achieved accomplishments as a child that I was quite proud of and felt went unnoticed. At the end of my Grade 5 semester, I was the only student invited back to dance, as the instructor recognized my potential. My parents were aware but had soon forgotten I was attending these extra classes and did not appear interested, or so it felt. And because I perceived they minimized my accomplishments, I began to minimize them myself. As a result, I lost interest and motivation in other opportunities, including the dance lessons. I neglected to cultivate these natural talents because I lacked the support and encouragement needed in order to feel confident and succeed.

My relationship with my parents had a profound effect on me, and because of this, it paved the way for attracting similar future relationships. Subconsciously, it taught me that the people in my life would also be short on encouragement and support. It taught me it would ultimately be all about them. And in looking back, it was.

My father was never encouraging or complimentary, only critical, telling me what I should be doing and not what a good job I had done. He was forever pointing out what was wrong instead of noticing what was right, always finding fault and error. Subsequently, the men in my life possessed the same critical nature and I subconsciously went in pursuit of them. Ultimately they would criticize my weight, my overall appearance, and, like my father, show little interest in my accomplishments.

I later learned these relationships were the very reasons that drove me to overeat. They were connected to the underlying reasons why I was stuffing down my emotions with food. I continued to attract and pursue these relationships with men until I was able to resolve these past issues with my father and permanently release the drive to overeat. This knowledge in itself was my liberation.

With this realization, I decided, for the last time, to try a completely different approach. Within a short period of time, using a rough semblance of what has now become the Method, I was able to work through these issues while mending my relationship with food. Had I not been able to find the root cause of my problem, I would never have overcome my struggle, enjoy healthy relationships, nor become the person I am today.

4

CHANGING YOUR SELF-TALK

Loving & Accepting Who You Are

When we let go of our critical inner voice,
we surrender ourselves to the unmistakable beauty
that lies within us all.

We unknowingly validate our negative beliefs with our own self-talk. We say, "I hate my thighs, my butt is too big, my arms are too fat, I'll never be skinny." And when we affirm negative beliefs long enough, we create self-fulfilling prophecies that, in turn, become our reality. If our belief is that we'll never look the way we want, then we never will.

We find it difficult accepting or acknowledging compliments because we assume others are thinking the same way as we feel about ourselves. Therefore, when given a compliment, we react with surprise and disbelief saying, "You really think that dress looks good on me? I think it makes me look fat." "You like my hair? I didn't think it looked that good. I was going to get it cut."

I believe people react to how we feel inside. If we have a belief about ourselves, negative or positive, then this is how others will treat us because this is the message we are projecting. We may feel unhappy with our weight, then find our spouse commenting on how we could afford to lose a few pounds or our mother telling us we shouldn't wear those pants because they make us look too fat.

I recall feeling this way and possessing many of these beliefs. One boyfriend said, "You know you're a big girl all over. You and I both know you're fat." At the impressionable age of 16, I unfortunately believed what he said. The words cut like a knife. I wondered how he could be so insensitive, but the reality was I had said the same thing to myself hundreds of times.

These are the self-fulfilling prophecies we create from the insecurities we have about our body image. They only serve to reinforce these beliefs and sadly, as a result, eventually begin to affect our actions. We find ourselves eating emotionally, turning to food for comfort, and struggling to keep the weight off. And we don't understand why this is happening. What we have done is create our own reality without even realizing it.

It's not surprising that we end up having such a negative attitude about ourselves. Using our own self-talk, we tell ourselves we're destined to be fat regardless of what we do, and no matter how much we exercise, we still don't like the way we look. We need to try harder because it's just not good enough. Imagine if you were to speak that way to children, how, over time, these comments would erode their self-esteem. But somehow we fail to recognize we're doing the same thing to ourselves, and we don't realize the impact it has on our self-image and our lives.

We often want to be something we're not because what we see is not good enough. Consequently, we overlook our own positive attributes. The grass always appears greener on the other side. We are envious of other people's appearance, health, happiness, or social standing, but the truth is, people are not without their share of problems. The secret is appreciating who we are and realizing our self-worth.

By refusing to accept ourselves, we're denying who we are, our true beauty. Instead, we berate ourselves, hating what we see, and feeling we have no self-control, which translates into the belief that we are a failure, unable to do anything right.

It is painfully evident by the way we speak to ourselves that we inevitably treat our bodies as though they are something to be loathed and not respected. Note the numerous times we put ourselves on a strict exercise program, and how unforgiving we were when it came to getting ourselves in shape. Instead of giving our body the love it needs, we inadvertently push it to the limit in our obsessive quest for unrealistic perfection. Working

out with weights one day, the ball the next, and numerous fitness classes in between, or running an inordinate
number of miles each day to increase our metabolism
and burn extra calories. We then end it all after falling weak to a craving, assaulting ourselves with sugary,
starchy, artery-clogging substances disguised as food.
They tax our heart, liver, and kidneys, which, in turn,
deplete our immune system, not to mention causing
foggy thinking and a real mean case of the sugar blues.

It is amazing really how our bodies have taken care of
us despite the abuse we've heaped upon them. This
becomes a dichotomy because, on the one hand,
you feel as though you're abusing yourself with food;
however, on the other hand, food is taking care of
you because it comforts you, it's your safe place. This
is how you nurtured and took care of yourself the
only way you knew how.

The next time we overeat and make the wrong
choices, we need not be so hard on ourselves. We
must think about how we would treat others in the
same situation. We can learn a lot about healing by

how we treat the ones we love when they need it most.

Visualization was a huge step in changing my core belief. It ultimately changed what I believed and consequently how I felt about myself. It changed how I looked at my life and responded to situations and interactions with others. Through visualization, loving and taking care of myself became natural for me without any conscious effort.

I would visualize situations where I felt self-conscious and insecure and then give myself love and encouragement. I discovered I had a strong desire to protect and take care of myself. I began to feel an intense love and compassion, and with this love and compassion came the healing I needed.

We need to love and accept our bodies just the way they are now. We can't hate ourselves and beat ourselves up and then expect to look beautiful. It doesn't work that way. Beauty does not respond to hate – it responds to love. And when we feel love, we radiate an inner beauty. If we hold our bodies in contempt, hating the way we look, the weight will remain unchanged. Our bodies are here to serve a purpose; they are here to take care of us and, in turn, we must love and take care of them.

I stood in front of the mirror and took a long, hard look at myself. What I was really looking at were all the years of abuse I had put my body through. I felt a momentary sadness and an overwhelming compassion to love and take care of it. It was a very moving experience, and this for me was a turning point, actually a starting point for the healing to begin.

It is interesting but sad how we so freely give others encouragement, patience, and love but are unable to give it to ourselves. When others are going through difficult times, we are right there giving them endless support, understanding, and kindness. How compassionate we are with them. When we show compassion toward others, imagine giving that same compassion and understanding to ourselves. Once we are able to do this, we will then find the road to healing not quite so long. Loving and accepting who we are enables us to let go of the weight we have long used for protection.

5

THE METHOD

Getting to the Root of the Problem

*All present problems are reminders
of what we haven't worked out in our past.*

Finding the root of our problem and resolving it eliminates the drive to overeat and allows us to let go of the ever-burdening weight that taxes our body, mind, and spirit. Using this Method frees us from the hold food has over us so that we can then move forward and live our lives the way they were meant to be lived.

I have formulated a Method based on various techniques used in overcoming my struggle with food. This Method will simply teach you how to find the root of your problem, work through it, and finally overcome it. I have successfully utilized it on my own, as well as with a partner.

Working With a Partner

Working with a partner may not only be beneficial in many ways, but for some, it may be the only way. Often when in the midst of a problem we become so involved and find it all-encompassing that we are unable to look at it objectively. The expression "It's easier to see the answer to someone else's problems when you're on the outside looking in," certainly holds merit in this situation. As a result, a partner will see things that we may overlook or are unaware of.

When we are inundated with problems that are troubling us, it can be beneficial to confide in a friend. Many of us who have joined a fitness club or walk together to stay fit already know the advantages of teamwork. The same holds true when you have a partner to support and encourage you.

When choosing a partner, bear in mind that it should be someone you trust and feel comfortable with in order to express yourself freely without fear of being judged, as this will allow you to speak openly and enable you to hear your own voice. In vocalizing your situation, what you are actually doing is putting your thoughts and concerns outside of yourself. When we do this, we begin to see our problems in a different light, allowing us to let go of the stress and frustration. It changes things and puts them into perspective and because of this, they don't seem to feel as enormous or overwhelming as we once believed.

A friend recently told me that she came to associate her problems with a large balloon. As she began to talk about them, it felt as though the balloon was gradually deflating so much so that she felt better able to handle them. She said, "I felt like I was letting go of all these negative emotions. It was like poison leaving my body."

Another equally important aspect of partnership is that it encourages you not only to make a commitment to yourself to follow through, but also makes you accountable to someone else. It is very convenient to make excuses and therefore procrastinate when there are issues we need to address.

Partnership further helps you to remain focused, enabling you to readily access the answers. It is surprising yet equally frustrating how easily our mind wanders, especially when trying to focus on issues we find difficult and often end up avoiding altogether. Your partner's help can be invaluable in guiding you through this process successfully by keeping your attention focused, as well as by giving you the needed encouragement and support only a friend can offer.

THE METHOD

1. Awareness of the Present Problem
2. Connect It to the Root of the Problem
3. Resolve It With a Visualization

1. Awareness of the Present Problem

It is important to become aware of problems that are presently bothering you because they are a direct connection to your cravings and overeating. Many times throughout the day we may encounter negative situations, but we need to be aware of the ones that particularly bother us and cannot be let go of. They are the ones we tend to ruminate over and relive. It could be something troubling you or a situation that leaves you feeling uncomfortable, fearful, or anxious. A co-worker who may make a nasty comment, a disagreement with a friend, or a rude stranger in line at the grocery store. Although some may say, "That's nothing, it happens all the time. How could this be causing me to overeat? Most people have things like this happen and they don't have this problem." You must remember that not everyone will react the same

57

to a situation. For some people, these occurrences simply roll off their back while others turn to food or equally destructive behaviours.

Often these present situations will not feel as though they are a direct link to your problem because there won't appear to be an obvious correlation. But once you begin working on them, you will notice how quickly your cravings disappear and how much you will feel in control. This Method will soon become second nature for you because it works.

When a Problem Becomes a Pattern

Many times a problem can go unrecognized because we fail to see the message it is conveying. If this problem is not dealt with, it will continue to occur until it becomes a pattern, happening over and over again. There could be a number of situations you may be experiencing – patterns of abusive relationships, continual involvement with pessimistic people, constantly being blamed for things that really aren't your fault, not being heard, or feeling you are a sounding board for someone's complaints as they chatter incessantly about themselves. Perhaps it's not being recognized for your attributes or others who neglect to build your self-esteem, belittling you in the process.

When we recognize a pattern, it enables us to open our eyes to a negative situation that is happening repeatedly. A boss or in-law who continuously talks down to us, an abusive husband or others who place high demands on us, making us feel it is our duty to carry the load. These are just a few examples of patterns that may occur in our lives, and they will continue to happen until we recognize them and work them out.

Most people experience patterns that occur throughout their entire lives, and often they go unnoticed, continuing to affect their quality of life. I had a tendency to attract the same type of men. Initially they appeared different from the rest; however, as the relationship progressed, I realized they all possessed the same glaringly negative traits. This problem was a long-standing pattern for many years until I learned how to recognize and resolve it.

Similarities in Past & Present Relationships

Some of the most profound relationships we experience are those that are close to our heart because they are more intense in nature. Often these complex relationships with parents, siblings, and close friends are at the root of our struggle with food, yet seldom do people make the connection between them.

If we take a closer look, we may see the similarity between the relationships in our past to those in our present. Interestingly, we tend to meet the same type of people who possess comparable personality traits and characteristics of those from our past. We need to recognize these similarities and, in doing so, they will help us identify and connect them back.

My father possessed a bad temper and could be aggressive and domineering; consequently, the men in my life were equally aggressive and domineering. It was just understood their actions were never to be questioned or challenged, as they were always right. Often I found myself trying to avoid rocking the boat.

It was no surprise that at that time I was at my heaviest and unable to control myself with food.

These unexplainable cravings and binges we experience are the result of the unresolved relationships that lie at the root of our problem. We must never underestimate the power and importance of our past because these first relationships tend to set the tone and therefore the pattern of the consequent relationships we experience throughout our lives.

Once you recognize the present problem, you can discern what it is telling you about yourself. Do you feel intimidated, humiliated, or insignificant? These are areas that need to be looked at and addressed. In essence, what you are doing is connecting them to issues or weaknesses you have experienced in your past and subconsciously held on to – times when you felt angry but weren't strong enough to stand up for yourself, times when you lacked confidence and were uncomfortable in your own skin. You will no longer be stuffing these emotions down with food.

When you crave and overeat, you feel as though you are completely out of control. But once you work through these areas, you will notice your cravings lose their sense of urgency. They will no longer have power over you.

Identify the Issue

We need to identify the issue in order to define exactly what is bothering us about a situation. This will enable us to effectively connect it to the root of our problem. The most important factor when identifying an issue is getting in touch with how you feel about it. I cannot stress the importance of this enough because these are your emotions and they are what drive you to crave and overeat.

You would begin by picturing or thinking about the present problem while asking yourself two important questions:

1. What specifically bothers me about this situation?
2. How does this make me feel?

Though these questions may seem obvious, it is imperative that you ask them, as they will allow you to look inward and identify the issue.

You may see that there are many different aspects of the problem you are able to look at. What you need to focus on is the one that affects you the most. You will know for sure when you get in touch with this feeling because it will be the part that immediately hits a nerve.

In order to identify the issue, I would picture or think about the incident. When asking myself *what bothered me about the situation*, I discovered:
"I felt taken advantage of and that my feelings didn't matter."

When I asked *how this made me feel*, a number of answers came to mind. I needed to choose the one that affected me the most, which was:
"I felt dominated and had to hold in my feelings."

Choosing this answer enabled me to identify the issue and exactly what was bothering me.

It is important at this point for you to write the answer down in order to remember it and connect it back to the root of the problem.

Use Your Own Words

When working with a partner, it is imperative that he or she help you "find your own words." When you are describing what it is that you're feeling, it will be your words, not your partner's that will help you connect it back.

While helping her friend Haley with a problem, Sara described Haley as a control freak but Haley described this feeling differently. In her own words, she expressed that she felt overwhelmed and burdened with responsibility. Looking at the varying differences of opinion, it is easy to see that if Haley had not used her own words, she never would have been able to connect this back to the root of her problem.

2. Connect It to the Root of the Problem

Now that you have identified exactly what it is that bothers you, you are ready to connect it to a similar incident from your past – the root of your problem. This incident must remind you of the present one and although it may not be exactly the same, it will *feel* the same. In order to do this, you need to recite the words you used and, while focusing on this, rephrase it into a question.

When I said that I felt dominated and had to hold in my feelings, I asked, "Who from my past was dominating, causing me to hold in my feelings?" Next, begin to think about the memories from your past; one will come to mind. Again, it may not be exactly the same, but it will *feel* the same.

This is an important step, as it will help you to accurately connect it to an earlier incident that reminds you of the present one. It may not necessarily be something that happened to you as far back as your childhood; rather, it may be something that happened several years ago or in your recent past.

While connecting this back, I began to scan memories from my past. In staying with this feeling, I was able to connect it to a similar feeling that was reminiscent of my father and the way he treated me as a child or, more clearly, the way I felt when I was with him. My father was volatile, and it did not take much before he would reach his breaking point. I was able to recollect many incidents from my past, but the one that stood out clearly was when I was 7 years old. I wanted my parents to get out of bed early one Saturday morning, so I stood in their bedroom saying, "Come on, Mommy, come on, Daddy, get up. It's time to wake up." They were unresponsive and continued to sleep, so I became more persistent. I was holding a pencil behind my back and, with both hands, slowly began bending it back and forth. I said, "If you don't get up, I'm going to break this pencil." At which point it accidentally snapped. My mother immediately disappeared out of the room while my father, in the midst of his rage, picked me up over his head and in his anger, threw me down on the bed numerous times, yelling and screaming. During this tirade I stiffened my body as a way to prevent being injured. I disconnected myself so as not to feel the physical pain. After my father stopped and left the room, I felt a calm relief that it was over and I was okay.

If anything, this one incident clearly outlined strict boundaries that taught me never to push my father, question him, or stand up to him. It also taught me to hold in my feelings. Incidents such as these did not happen too often because I quickly learned the rules. Although both incidents appeared completely different from an outside perspective, they both felt the same.

What If I Recall More Than One Incident From My Past?

If more than one incident comes to mind, ask yourself which one affects you the most. It will be the one that you have the strongest connection to and the strongest emotions around.

What If I'm Unable to Find an Incident From My Past?

Some problems are easier to connect back than others, but occasionally we may not be able to find an incident or person from our past. If this happens, I recommend visualizing the present incident. The connection will come to you while you are visualizing it or at a later time, but be assured you will find the connection.

Write It Down

Once you have found the connection to the root of your problem, it is of the utmost importance to write it down because, more often than not, it is forgotten. We may not always have time to work on it at that exact moment; therefore, when we do have the time, we will know what it is that needs to be done. I like to put my notes by my bedside and work on them before going to sleep.

Assessing the Root of the Problem

Now that you have connected the issue to the root of your problem, you are ready to look at it from an outside perspective. The reason for this is so that you will be able to understand more about the situation and assess which part is logical and which part is emotional. Whenever I thought about breaking the pencil, it was always from a highly emotional standpoint, but looking at it from an outside perspective, I was able to assess the situation logically and rationally.

I realized my father's need to always be right and unquestioned. Looking back, I could see his behaviour stemmed from his own fears and insecurities. When he would become angry with us, I was much too fearful of the impending repercussions to question him and therefore remained quiet. The truth was, I never felt his actions were appropriate or warranted. I also realized my father lost his temper because he did not know how to handle our misbehaviour. He was born and raised at a time when children were expected to do as they were told, without question, and consequently this was the belief he bestowed upon his own children. He did not feel he needed to answer to us or explain himself and was unaware of the effect his actions would have on us later in life.

Looking back, I could see just how much his anger alone affected me. Without realizing it, I continued to attract men with the same temperament and domineering traits. During this time, I dealt with it in the only way familiar to me, which was to turn my dependency toward food, where I found solace.

Understanding why others behave the way they do is an important part of the healing process. With this understanding comes compassion, and once compassion is felt we can then let go of the anger and resentment we have been holding on to. When we look at the incident from an outside perspective, we are able to see it for what it really is, enabling us to let go of the emotional hold it has on our lives.

3. Resolve It With a Visualization

Visualization is a vital component of the Method, as it enables us to work out unresolved issues at the root of our problem. It gives us the opportunity to resolve these issues, releasing buried emotions that have been suppressed for many years.

Visualization will give you a chance to change the negative beliefs that have influenced you throughout your life. The end result will leave you a more positive individual minus an emotional dependence on food. I have touched lightly on this here; however, it is fully explained in the next chapter on visualization.

Visualization is essentially the same as daydreaming. It is the same as picturing something you have experienced. Similarly, when we are relaying a story and describing it, we are visualizing. As we visualize, we will find that more information is revealed to us about an experience, which will help to further resolve the issue. You may choose to visualize the incident or visualize the person in order to speak to him or her on neutral ground. If you were physically attacked, you would not want to visualize the attack itself, but instead picture yourself with that person in a safe place.

How to Visualize

Choose a time and a quiet place where you are best able to focus. Sit in a comfortable chair. With eyes closed, relax your body and quiet your mind. I find the best time is just before I fall asleep. It is a good way to work out troubling issues that arise throughout the day and also a powerfully effective way for me to end my day. Regardless of when you choose to do this, it is imperative you set aside the time. To begin, think about the person you want to talk to and imagine him in front of you. Feel free to let out all your emotions; just go with whatever arises. You may want to ask why he did what he did as this is an important part of the healing process. Just wait patiently for the answer, he will tell you. Trust what you hear is right, that it's real for you. You may even be surprised at what you hear. Remember, much of visualization is trusting yourself. The rest will come easily. This is further explained in the next chapter.

With visualization, I was able to let out the anger and fear I had been holding onto for years. I told my father how his aggressive behaviour had a profound effect on my life and how I suffered from the repercussions. When he realized this, I could see and feel the pain and remorse he felt. I

asked him questions that helped me understand
his fears and why he did the things he did. This
was an immeasurable release for me. I never realized just how much energy was spent holding
on to all this stress and tension. I felt an inner
strength surface. This visualization allowed me to
see things clearly, enabling me to let go of the
hurt and pain.

It was not long before I noticed that the pattern of
attracting aggressive and domineering men into my
life stopped. The need to turn to food lessened considerably as I now felt more whole.

As we resolve each situation that is connected to our
problem, our cravings and overeating will come to
an end.

Going Back to an Incident More Than Once

There will be times when you want to visualize an
incident more than once if you feel it has not been
fully resolved. This is to ensure you have said everything you need to say or ask. You might find it too

much to accomplish all at once; therefore, this gradual process may be easier for you.

For example, the first time you visualize an incident, you may just want to express your emotions. The next time, you might ask why he treated you this way and conclude by giving him a gift of your wisdom and knowledge. This is further addressed in the next chapter.

How Will I Know When an Incident is Resolved?

You will know an incident is resolved because, when you think about it, it will no longer bother you. You will also experience a release and a feeling of calm, bringing you to a place of forgiveness.

Resolving Different Parts of an Incident

There were a number of times I would visualize the same incident when working on issues concerning my father, as there were various aspects I still needed to complete. Sometimes you will notice that the same incident will bother you, even though you were sure you had already worked it out. In actuality, you have worked it out. What you are experiencing is a different part of the problem, another piece of the puzzle, and therefore one you will want to address.

Recently a friend I had previously helped with a problem concerning her daughter approached me about another issue she was having. Using my Method we connected it back to an incident 30 years prior, and, to her annoyance, she found herself in the same situation again concerning her mother. Frustrated, she said, "I've already worked on that. Why do I have to work on that again?" I explained that this was a different part of the problem. Where it previously had been a power struggle, she now felt cornered and helpless. My friend was relieved to see that this was a different part of the problem and felt confident she could completely resolve it.

Even though we may find ourselves back in the same situation again with any number of emotions – feeling isolated, unloved, or even dominated, we can be assured that once we resolve them, they will no longer need to be addressed.

Visualization is invaluable, as it will help you to let go of your emotional attachment to these issues. In overcoming this, you will feel the joy of experiencing life in a more secure, open, and loving way. When we visualize and give the inner child within us the strength, courage, and support required, this then will instill these same attributes within ourselves. And with these attributes, we will imbue self-worth, and this positive effect will carry over into our present lives.

I firmly believe our present problems are reminders of what we have not worked out in our past, and what we have not worked out we often tend to deal with by overeating.

Once we resolve the root of our problem, we will experience a feeling of freedom – freedom from the negative reoccurring incidents and freedom from the cravings, overeating, and constant suffering that have held us captive. And in return, we will be given a precious gift, a gift of the knowledge that once we experience this freedom, it will be ours to hold without fear of ever relinquishing it to our past.

The Method at a Glance

1. **Awareness of the Present Problem.**

   Ask yourself what is presently bothering you.

2. **Connect It to the Root of the Problem.**

   Once you identify the problem, focus on your past to find the connection. Write it down.

3. **Resolve It With a Visualization.**

   Visualize the person and express your emotions.

6

VISUALIZATION

....

It's Easier Than You Think

*Visualization is an entirely personal experience,
as each person will walk away with
his or her own interpretation.*

People tend to avoid visualization feeling it is time
consuming, overwhelming, or that it is just too difficult. To this end I have formulated a simple, easy to
follow technique that can be accomplished in as little
as ten to fifteen minutes. In my attempt to answer

the most commonly asked questions, I have chosen to devote an entire chapter on it.

How Is Visualization Going to Stop Me From Overeating? How Do I Know It's Going to Make a Difference?

Visualization works to affect change within us, and once this change has occurred, our struggle with food will end. We carry around excess stress and tension from unresolved issues, both in our past and present. Our body holds fast to these issues and they are what drive us to crave and overeat.

If you had the opportunity to travel back in time and say what you've always wanted to say and make things right, wouldn't you? And by doing so, you could rid yourself of stress, tension, and all related problems – would you not jump at the chance? Of course you would – we all would. And in releasing all that stress and tension, our bodies would enter a state of calm allowing us to relax in a way we have long forgotten.

Visualization does just that. It gives us a chance to overcome past experiences we believed we were powerless over, providing us with the opportunity to finally make it right. Visualization stops the drive to crave and overeat because the need to eat due to stress and tension will no longer be there.

What Is Visualization?

Visualization is easier than you think. It is the same as daydreaming, thinking back to a past experience. Imagine for a moment your mind wandering off, thinking about your morning, taking a shower, getting dressed, and eating breakfast. That is visualization. Often we find ourselves daydreaming, whether we're caught in traffic, sitting at our desk, or going for a run. When we daydream, we are visualizing, it is one in the same.

What if I'm Unable to Visualize?

Many people believe that when they visualize, they should see actual pictures in their mind. This, however, is not always the case, as there are those who experience a feeling or a sense of the situation.

How Long Does It Take to Do a Visualization?

Visualization can take as little as 10 to 15 minutes. You will be surprised at what you can accomplish in such a short amount of time. I will often spend 10 minutes with a visualization; however, sometimes I will spend up to 30 minutes on one. When you look at all the years wasted battling with your weight, in comparison, the time invested in visualization is minimal.

When Should I Do a Visualization?

The most effective time to do a visualization will be determined by your own schedule. For some, the first few moments upon awakening are preferable, while for others, the best time is just before they fall asleep.

How Will Visualization Empower Me?

Often when we think back to a negative situation, usually our focus is on how overpowering it was, making us feel weak and vulnerable. Sadly, it is our nature as humans to direct our thoughts toward fears and weaknesses instead of our strengths and abilities.

When we visualize, we are able to look at a situation from a broader perspective, enabling us to recognize our unrealized strengths, thereby putting them into action.

How Can I Be Sure What I Remember Is Accurate?

How can we be sure what we remember is the truth, that it actually happened? This is a question many of us may have when recalling a past incident. Whether it's entirely accurate or not does not matter. It is what you remember and have believed to be true all these years because this is what you have been building your life upon. Don't go by someone else's recollection because that is their memory, not yours. You have to go by your own because it is your truth.

A friend confided that at an early age she became fearful of her mother dying. Monika recalled overhearing a conversation her mother was engaged in, stating should anything happen to her, the children would be sent off to live with relatives. The thought of losing her mother and having her world torn apart marked the beginning of this unrealistic fear. When asked years later, her older siblings replied that to their knowledge no mention of this was ever made. Monika began to doubt the validity of what she had heard many years ago but realized that true or not this was her memory and one she had built her life upon.

What Could I Possibly Accomplish by Having to Revisit This Experience Again?

When we visualize an experience, it is natural to question why we need to speak to this person again when what he or she did was unforgivable. It is important to revisit this experience because it enables us to release pent-up feelings that are detrimental not only to our psychological health but also our physical well-being, as evident in the many ailments that have become commonplace today.

What If I'm Afraid to Look Back?

Many of us, if we are being honest with ourselves, avoid situations because of fear. When we refuse to face something, it becomes a much larger and decidedly more ominous problem. Ultimately this gives it more power and control than it actually has. Just the mere fact that we avoid it, gives it power. We may think if we visualize something from our past, we will only be dragging up painful memories. We might ask why we would want to subject ourselves to that again, remembering only too well how it felt. However, when we visualize, we give ourselves the opportunity to see things not only from a safe place but also from a better and stronger position.

Looking at a situation from a different perspective in time relinquishes the power and hold it has over us. It may surprise us to find that in looking back, it wasn't as bad as previously thought and that we handled it much better than we realized. It is important to keep in mind that this is a memory. We are in the present, in control, and can therefore face it without fear of being hurt.

When strong emotions are involved, a situation can often seem worse than it actually is. Our perception may be distorted from the hurt and pain we experienced, but when we visualize, we are able to see it with clarity. At the age of 7 I was bullied at school and, looking back, always felt hurt and sorry for myself. I remembered thinking how cruel and unfeeling these children were. But with visualization I realized just how strong I was and how well I handled the situation. I was able to see that I possessed a strength and maturity well beyond my years. Visualization was key in taking away the power these upsetting memories held for me.

When we visualize, we are able to change how we feel about a situation because we are looking through wiser and more experienced eyes with a proportionately deeper understanding and knowledge.

With maturity comes the ability
to transform and strengthen who we once were.

How Can I Get Through to Someone Who Has Hurt Me?

When you speak to someone during a visualization, you must speak to her past her guard, past her ego. You will do this not by looking at her but by looking into her, into her mind, her vulnerable side, the very core and pureness of who she is. Speak to that quiet, peaceful, reflective place inside. You now have the opportunity to see and understand who she really is and realize her fears and pain. You may discover that underneath her many layers of protection, what she really wanted was love and acceptance. Unfortunately she went about it the wrong way.

Speaking to her very core will help her realize and understand the damage caused as a result of her behaviour. At this point, you will then find her open and accepting to what you have to say.

During a Visualization, How Can I Be Sure the Other Person's Response Is True? How Do I Know I'm Not Making It Up?

When asking someone a question, make sure the person is speaking from her heart. While looking into her, you will be able to feel how she is feeling. If she has her guard up and is not speaking from her heart, you will know. Learn to trust yourself with this.

Why Visualization?
Why Not Confront the Person?

Visualization is more effective because under normal circumstances a heated argument could ensue, causing walls to go up, cutting off communication. We need to address the relationship with this person, in the past, where the problem originated, not in the present, as the dynamics have now changed. Visualization is a fast and successful technique that enables you to speak to someone by bypassing any barriers he or she would normally put up. Without visualization this would be virtually impossible, as the risk of further damaging the relationship and alienating yourself would be unavoidable.

What If I Could Never Imagine Feeling Compassion for This Person?

You may believe that you could never imagine feeling compassion, and, if you could, how would this help you feel better about what happened? Julie's experience comes to mind as a perfect example of anger melting into compassion.

"I was late one morning for an important meeting and found myself stuck behind a slow-moving vehicle. I started to become agitated and felt my blood pressure rise and my heart race. There was a pain in the back of my neck and I thought my temper was going to blow through the roof. I wondered what kind of moron drives at this speed. He was obviously not paying attention or he would have seen that I was almost on top of him. Finally there was an opening further ahead and I was able to pass. I could hardly wait to give him a dirty look that would make him realize how inconsiderate and self-absorbed he was. Just as I began to pass the car, it slowly moved off onto the shoulder of the road. I was able to see that inside was an elderly man and his wife and realized they were in trouble. As I stopped to offer assistance, I immediately felt the anger and the pain in my neck subside. As it turned out, his wife was ill and he was trying to help her until he could safely pull over."

Julie was glad to be of help to these people, but more importantly she was able to understand why this man was driving the way he was. By the time she realized what had happened, she no longer felt anger, only under-standing and compassion. Once we truly understand someone it is then that we are able to feel compassion.

What Will I Hope to Accomplish by Gaining Understanding and Compassion?

As hard as it is to imagine, understanding and com-passion will free you from the negative emotions you have been holding on to and bring you to a place of peace. Like most people, we don't want to feel these emotions because of the pain they cause us, so without even realizing it, we stuff them down with food.

If we were to look at Julie, it would be easy to see that she was frustrated and angered stuck behind this car. Once her anger and frustration dissipated, she was able to continue with her day and focus on other things rather than carry around this stress. Imagine how exhausting and how much energy, holding on to all this tension, would take. We won-der why we have back problems, stomach problems, and other health issues. With compassion comes forgiveness, and it is forgiveness that will allow you to let go, freeing you from the drive to crave and overeat.

The Steps to Visualization

For those of you who already make visualization an important part of your day, you may prefer to do this while going for a run or exercising. Although the standard recommendation for visualization is sitting quietly with closed eyes, there are many who find it just as effective while engaging in other activities. Of course, you must bear in mind the safety precautions, as some activities require your full attention. Following the steps below will ensure success.

Visualization on Your Own

1. To begin, either sit or lie in a quiet, comfortable place and close your eyes. Take a deep breath and clear your mind of all present issues. Relax your body, starting from your feet and continue with your calves, thighs, hips, stomach, lower back, hands, arms, chest, neck, face, and head.

2. Once you feel relaxed, think back to the incident from your past or, if you prefer, you may just visualize the person with whom you wish to speak.

3. You may either want to let out your anger and frustration or simply speak to the person. If the latter is the case, then you must speak past his guard, into his vulnerable side, by looking into him, his very core. Speak to that quiet, reflective place in his mind.

4. You are now able to see and understand who he really is. Notice his fears and pain.

5. Talk about the way he treated you and convey how it felt. But most importantly, express the effect it had on you and how it impacted your life.

6. Be sure he understands your pain. You will know he sincerely feels it because something in him will change. You might sense a softness in him, he may exhibit sadness and remorse, or he may give in to his emotions.

7. Ask why he behaved the way he did and listen for his response. You will either hear his

answer or you will feel or sense it. Every visualization is different and unique.

8. Once you have heard or sensed his response, you would then give him a gift, a gift imparting your wisdom and knowledge, to help him realize the result of his actions and show him a better way; that if he had done things differently, how wonderful his life could be. This will create a shift or a change in the way both sides feel and you may experience a form of release. This is effective regardless of whether or not the person is living or deceased.

9. If you are not ready to forgive and have not yet come to a place of understanding and compassion, then you may choose to continue this visualization at another time until you have said everything you need to say. Sometimes we need to review or assimilate one part of the issue at a time in order to move on to the next. If, however, you are ready to forgive, then you can communicate this to him now. Bear in mind, forgiveness

cannot occur until understanding and compassion are felt.

10. Take a deep breath, relax your body, and slowly open your eyes or you may just naturally fall asleep.

11. If an earlier memory comes up for you during or after your visualization, then go to the earlier one and visualize it. You may find that there is still more to be worked out at an even deeper level.

Visualization With a Partner

1. You can guide your partner following the steps from "Visualization on Your Own."

2. While your partner is visualizing, it is best that she vocalizes in her mind, although, if she prefers, she can speak out loud. Regardless of which way she chooses, you will still need to be there to follow along with her as the conversation transpires and guide her through it. Her eyes should remain closed.

3. Guide your partner in either one of the two approaches used above in step #3 of "Visualization on Your Own."

4. Make sure your partner is able to see and understand who the person, she is visualizing, really is. Have her notice his or her fears and pain.

5. If your partner chooses to remain silent during the visualization, have her tell you what has transpired after each part of the conversation so that you can follow along and assist her. You might ask if she senses or feels anything from that person.

6. If your partner becomes stuck on an incident, give her suggestions on what she can say or ask. Help her through it.

7. Most importantly, have your partner give this person a gift, a gift imparting her wisdom and knowledge. (Review step #8 of "Visualization on Your Own.") This will create a change or a shift in the way both sides feel and your partner may experience a form of release.

This is effective regardless of whether or not the person is living or deceased.

8. If your partner has an earlier memory that comes up for her during or after the visualization, have her go to the earlier one and visualize it as she may find that there is still more to be worked out at an even deeper level.

Other Visualization Techniques

Below I have listed other techniques to support and assist you with your visualizations.

Technique #1
Supporting the Child Within You

When visualizing yourself in a past incident, as a child, you would enter the visualization as your adult self and join the child. You can now assist yourself (the child) when speaking to the person you need to confront. The importance of this is so that you, as the child, feel the support and protection from your adult self.

Technique #2

Visualizing From an Outside Perspective

During a visualization, rather than placing yourself inside the situation, observe it from an outside perspective by placing yourself in the audience of a theatre and watching it unfold onstage. Many people embrace this type of visualization from a distance because they find it more comfortable.

Technique #3

Asking for Help & Support

While visualizing, you can ask for help and support from someone you trust and admire, such as a mentor, to guide you with his or her wisdom and good judgment. This is helpful, as it can give you insight into a situation and allow you to see things from a new perspective.

Journaling

After a visualization you may find it beneficial to journal about your experience. Writing it down helps put together everything you have learned, as well as any realizations you have made. It further assists in helping you make new connections to other past incidents. As you visualize, you move closer to completely resolving the root of your overeating. Journaling your thoughts, feelings, and experiences will inevitably move you one step closer toward the healing process.

7

Always Say Yes

....

A Technique That Allows You to Eat What You Want & Still Lose Weight

The following guidelines are in no way meant to replace medical advice. Before embarking on any dietary changes or programs, it is advisable to check with your doctor first.

This technique will prevent you from overeating and succumbing to your cravings, yet still allow you to eat the foods you enjoy. It proved to be not only a life-saver for me, as I lost weight and was able to eat what

I wanted without feeling deprived, but also invaluable, as it helped me remain in control.

This technique will ensure
long-term successful weight loss
without the fear of craving and overeating.

The guidelines I have listed below will help you develop a routine enabling you to create structure and organization in your life regardless of where you are or what you are doing.

A Word About Snacks

There are two different schools of thought on this. Snacking throughout the day will keep your blood sugar levels up, preventing you from making unhealthy choices. On the other hand, your taste buds are kept stimulated, causing cravings that make it difficult to abstain. Some find by snacking they are unable to recognize whether or not they are truly hungry. It is important to recognize true hunger so that when you do eat, you will know when you feel satisfied. This will help teach you to fully appreciate each meal.

Do Not Diet

While working on the root of your problem, I recommend that you do not diet. If you are dieting, you are restricting yourself. And when we restrict ourselves, we crave, which results in overeating. Whatever we can't have, we want all the more.

This technique allows you to eat the food you crave without ever having to diet.

The Technique

When I experienced a craving, using the technique, I would tell myself, "Yes, I can have it either at my next meal or meal of choice." This would then be consumed with that meal and not as a snack.

The secret... I was saying "yes" to myself. Psychologically, when we say no, we want it more. When we say yes, however, something in our mind changes and we find we can easily hold off until our next meal. This works because we are the one making the decision, we are taking control. As a result of saying yes, I never felt deprived because I never refused or denied myself anything I craved. This technique was effortless for me.

When we say no to a craving,
the struggle & temptation escalate to unwanted heights.
Saying yes gives us back our power.

At dinner I would have a lighter meal and then afterward eat what I had set aside. In doing this, I was not consuming unwanted calories and at the same time was satisfying my craving. Often the unexpected would happen; I no longer wanted it, as the desire had passed. It was liberating to know I could have what I wanted, and this knowledge alone released a tremendous amount of pressure off me.

It is important to satisfy our cravings,
not fill up on food we don't really want.

Nighttime Eating

Experts agree that we should not eat in the evening when attempting to lose or maintain our weight. It is easy to become accustomed to nighttime eating because at the end of our day, when we begin to unwind and relax, we often seek comfort in the form of food. It's always there. It never lets us down and far too often becomes a habit, a dangerous replacement for other activities. When we succumb to these late night cravings, not only are we unable to fend them off but also spending an evening without eating will become an impossibility.

I have spoken to many people who discovered that when they ate in the evening, the following night would find them strongly craving comfort food, high in fat and sugar. However, when they did not eat during the evening for a few days, their cravings subsided as they lost the urge to eat at that time.

What To Do During the Evening

During the evening I would often make myself a cup of hot chocolate. This would satisfy my desire for something sweet and flavourful, and the warmth of the milk was comforting and filling. A friend told me that drinking hot chocolate at night was the one thing that helped her get through the difficult cravings. For those who prefer something different, another alternative might be Chai tea with honey and milk.

What to Drink

Studies show we should drink at least six to eight glasses of water per day to keep hydrated and flush toxins from our body.

How to Increase Your Metabolism

Visualization has been very effective in increasing my metabolism. While eating a meal, I would affirm, "My metabolism is speeding up. I feel the food digesting quickly. I feel myself getting thinner." I would then visualize and feel this happening. I noticed results shortly thereafter. You can also target a specific area of your body by focusing your attention on it as you visualize it becoming smaller.

What to Do When Feeling Bored, Restless, or Stressed and Find Yourself Craving

Often when we feel any number of emotions, we deal with them by overindulging in an attempt to appease ourselves. Whenever I felt any of these emotions I would visualize and affirm, "When I'm feeling bored, restless, stressed, I have no desire to eat. I have no appetite when I'm feeling this way." I would then visualize feeling the physical sensation of losing my appetite. Whatever feeling that is, whether it is a feeling of excitement or an energized feeling in the core area of your body, you need to focus on that sensation. With practice, you will become proficient at changing your association when these emotions arise and you will automatically lose your appetite.

Negative Self-Talk

Be aware of negative self-talk; it is dangerous and counter productive and we are all experts at perpetuating it. When you find yourself saying that your struggle with weight loss has been far too difficult and is just not working, remember, this is your negative self-talk. And this self-destructive talk has been a roadblock standing in your way, immobilizing you. In order to move beyond this, you need to visualize and focus on what you desire, your intention. Visualization will be the one important component in conquering your negative self-talk when used in this way.

When I followed this technique while working on the root of my overeating, I was able to lose weight and still enjoy what I loved without feeling deprived or fearful of gaining it back. It liberated me from feeling out of control or confined within the walls of a diet I was unwilling to commit to. It restored my faith and I began to see a positive change in myself.

8

At Last…Freedom

*How It Felt to Overcome
My Struggle With Food*

*Getting to the root of your overeating
will leave you feeling more in control, more positive,
more at ease, and infinitely more at peace.*

Overcoming my struggle with food began as a subtle, gradual, yet powerful change, though when it was over, I knew without a doubt it had ended. It was a quiet knowledge, a feeling of finality that it was gone for good. This I knew, as it was a self-assuredness I had never experienced before. I used to dream of the day that this raging storm would stop but I never imagined it to happen this way.

I began to notice that the all too familiar nagging, tormenting feelings were lessening until gradually they became nonexistent. The evening hours always seemed to bring about their own particular brand of hell, but that, too, was changing as I found I no longer had the urge to eat into the early hours of the morning.

The urgency to put myself on yet another diet ceased as I noticed that I began to lose weight without trying. The feelings of deprivation diminished as I began to eat more well-balanced meals. When others were eating food that I normally agonized over, I found I no longer had the urge to dive in. The lifelong storm had now abated.

When I did enjoy something I craved, it was easy to stop once I was satisfied. The secret was knowing I could have it whenever I wanted. Gone were the urges and cravings for more. The fear that food would set me off on another eating tangent as it had done in the past no longer consumed my every thought. Not only did I not gain weight, but also the psychological torture I put myself through no longer accompanied it. As a result, I was able to turn my focus to other interests that had long taken a back seat to this demon.

The erratic roller-coaster of emotional highs and lows I had become accustomed to stabilized, and I felt more present, more conscious, without thoughts of food tormenting me. I now had my power back and this gave me a calm sense of control. It was as though I had awoken from a hazy, dreamlike state. My senses became more acute, my thoughts and emotions clearer. Looking around, I began to notice things outside myself because until then I had been so inwardly focused.

My relationship with those closest to me improved, and out of this emerged a greater sense of belonging. I was able to truly appreciate their presence in my life, as well as the happiness they brought. A newfound peace and serenity now resided within that had long been absent. I had come home to stay – this time for good.

If I were asked to describe how my life is now, how I feel as a result of overcoming this struggle, I would begin with one word – freedom. Freedom from craving and overeating, freedom from obsessing and plotting to get more, and freedom from the remorse over not being able to stop. Relief, happiness, and increased self-esteem are just a few others that come to mind.

I look at myself now and realize how amazing it is to live each day no longer having food constantly nagging at me. At the same time, I can't help but be painfully aware that a large percentage of the population still constantly struggles with this, many going through the torment that once was a way of life for me. If there were an opportunity for me to give back, to help others, now was the time to do it.

It has become a constant daily reminder how truly effective and permanent this Method really is. Twenty-five years ago when I embarked on this path to recovery, I had no idea the impact this would have on my future and consequently on the future of others that I would ultimately help.

It is a completely liberating feeling to know that I can eat all those sinfully, decadent, forbidden foods that in the past tortured me. Even after having these foods in moderation, I am able to continue on without all the obsessive thoughts. Ice cream, chips, and dessert are no longer a threat because now there is no fear of losing control.

I appreciate and admire my appearance each and every day in contrast with how much I had hated myself and how I looked. And, as a result, I have developed a positive body image. Throughout the time that I was overcoming my problem with food, I realized I had come to love who I was. It really was a new awakening for me, and this awakening has been consistent for the past 25 years.

My energy levels improved considerably, and I no longer had that lethargic and bloated feeling due to the overeating and weight gain. Gone were the carb hangovers that had become a common occurrence. And when I worked out, I could see results. I felt I was able to sculpt my body, whereas in the past this was not only difficult but next to impossible.

It was an incredible relief to be able to concentrate on other areas of interest without my mind wandering off to think about food. Until then, it felt as though the mental struggle and the cravings were holding me back. I had always planned to take a course or pursue a career once I got my cravings and overeating under control. Now that I had resolved this, I was able to move forward.

I was relieved to no longer live a double life, hiding what I was thinking, feeling, and planning. Always plotting to get two or three more pieces of cake while trying to figure out ways I could do this without being revealed. I recall, when at parties or special occasions, I always had the feeling I was committing some sort of crime as I would sneak around stealing unwanted desserts from other people's plates. It was reminiscent of the Seinfeld episode in which George

Costanza takes the untouched chocolate éclair out of the garbage and eats it. The biggest part of overcoming this problem was knowing that I never had to deal with or experience these issues again.

With the success of this Method, my weight has been consistent, and although there are days when I eat the wrong foods, I enjoy every bite without the guilt. I don't want to live a strict, regimented life where I feel I have to be ever vigilant about everything I put onto my plate and into my mouth.

Throughout the subsequent 25 years, I have used this Method to help myself in other areas of life and continue to do so today. It was created not only to help others find and resolve the root of their overeating, but also enable them to apply it to their own life where there is a desire to make a permanent change. My belief is that once the connection is found, then the healing can begin.

9

LAUREN'S STORY

To be free from the destructive beliefs
we have about ourselves
opens the door to change, allowing us to step
through, leaving behind our skin of self-doubt.

I believe most things in life happen for a reason, and I believe we meet the people we are destined to meet. Making Lauren's acquaintance was, to my mind, a fortunate accident, as I happened to be at my local health food store at a time of day that was highly unusual for me. Lauren was helping me choose an appropriate vitamin supplement when our conversation turned to the topic of stress and the effect it has on us. In discussing the many different ways people react to stress, some turning to alcohol, others to drugs, I learned that for Lauren it was food.

Lauren admitted that at the age of 15 her weight tipped the scales at 225. Painfully aware she was eating when not even hungry, Lauren remained frustrated because she could not understand her inability to control herself. One of the many well-intentioned suggestions Lauren received was to express herself through artistic means, in her case, music. Not surprisingly, it was unsuccessful, as it failed to address the reason why she was overeating. Now at 23, her weight hovers at 195 and she feels unstable because of her fear of gaining it all back.

I realized Lauren would benefit from learning the Method and was pleased at how open she was to the concept and how well she understood it. I told her that once the connection is found and resolved at the root her problem, the drive to overeat would be gone for good. I assured her that, like me, she would feel completely in control of her life and never have to put herself on another diet. Lauren recalled walking home from work that evening as she thought of the many memories of her past and felt excited and hopeful that she now had the ability to work through these issues.

Over the course of the next few weeks, Lauren and I settled into an easy, comfortable friendship. We talked about her progress toward finding the root of her problem. She asked many questions to further her understanding of the Method and to perfect it. Being with Lauren reminded me of myself and how willing and unafraid I was to try new and unfamiliar concepts. Lauren proved to be a quick study. She became adept at applying the Method and noticed her cravings subsiding. Lauren's determination and commitment left me confident that it would only be a matter of time before she would overcome this.

Lauren confided in me about a traumatic incident from her past that she was unable to free herself from. She was assaulted at the age of 17 by a man, she recalls, seemed friendly enough. Lauren had been out for the evening with a friend when a misunderstanding took place, leaving her without money or transportation. During her attempt to find a way home, she met a man who invited her back to his apartment for a few drinks on the pretense he had money there to give her for a bus ticket or cab. Lauren innocently went with him. After a few drinks, she was unable to move her arms or legs. She could not even speak. Lauren had been drugged.

The physical assault alone was horrible, but the verbal abuse that followed was in many ways worse. The cruel and demeaning comments cut to the core. She carried this memory and his words with her for so long that she came to believe them. Lauren told no one because of the humiliation and blame she felt for putting herself in this situation. There wasn't a day that went by she did not in some way relive it. Not long after the attack, Lauren remembers sitting alone on a park bench repeating over and over, "Erase this memory! Erase this memory!" No matter how much she begged and prayed for it to go away, it never did.

Lauren said, "For rape, they give a man seven years, but for the victim it's a lifetime sentence."

Lauren often felt anger toward anyone who showed her kindness and love. She realized she was becoming cynical in her belief that any act of kindness concealed a motive for selfish gain. She hated that she felt this way. Because of her inability to accept love and kindness, she was left feeling guarded and afraid. Unknowingly, Lauren put up a barrier, preventing her from truly experiencing all that life had to offer. It was a form of protection from being physically and emotionally raped again. Food had also become a safeguard, and the added weight helped insulate her from the outside world.

We talked about why she was holding on to these beliefs and why she had allowed this man's words to become her truth. I helped her understand that these hurtful comments imposed upon her were untrue and weren't about her – they were about him, his life. She began to see the truth in this. Lauren remembered this man's apartment, which had a bare and empty look. There was nothing but a few pieces of furniture. There were no pictures, no memories, or sentiments. He was a lost soul without connections, family, or friends. There was an anger in him and a desire to take it out on the world, in this case an innocent, trusting, young girl. I told Lauren that visualization was the key to resolving this so she could be free from the memory.

Lauren, feeling ready to do a visualization, finally decided to confront this man. She was somewhat apprehensive because whenever she thought about that night it would upset her, bringing forth a flood of emotions she would stuff back down with food. Lauren now realized that she would be facing him without food to buffer her fall.

Lauren was able to let go of all her pent-up anger and pain. But in order to completely overcome this, she needed to first understand her assailant. On the surface, she saw intense anger and frustration, but underneath she sensed an emptiness deep down inside that was completely numb. She felt that even deeper, there was a great loneliness. She could see a desperation, the need for human touch, but the only way he knew how was through force. In understanding him, Lauren was surprised to see her focus had shifted, no longer on her own pain, but now on his. She was able through this understanding to find her own strength and courage to feel compassion for this man. Lauren came to fully understand and experience through this visualization the power of forgiveness. What an amazing breakthrough!

The next morning, however, Lauren was disappointed with the array of negative emotions she was feeling, especially after the powerful visualization she experienced the night before. She was feeling unloved and unworthy. In identifying her feelings, Lauren was able to remember that she had felt this way as a young child. In using the Method, it enabled Lauren to connect this to her father, the root of her problem.

Lauren remembered that her problems began at the age of 6, with the death of her grandfather. He suffered from alcoholism, and for many years Lauren's father recalls his youth being peppered with episodes of mental and physical abuse. Lauren's father spent most of his life trying to live up to his father's expectations. He eventually lost touch with himself and his aspirations and, as a result, became an angry, frustrated, bitter man. With this came the physical and emotional abuse. Lauren remembers the beatings. Her evening prayers consisted of pleas to let her go and live with God in heaven. She would awake in the morning, feeling sad and disappointed that she was still there.

Lauren believed her father looked at her as stupid and clumsy, that there was something wrong with her. Recalling when a mistake was made, he would say, "Oh, looks like a Lauren." This comment only reinforced her belief that she was stupid and couldn't do anything right. As a result, Lauren developed low self-esteem and felt being mistreated was acceptable because, as she put it, "I'm not worth it, anyway." She also believed if something good were to happen, it would be short-lived because she didn't deserve it.

By the time Lauren was 12 years old, she unknowingly learned to repress her emotions by stuffing them down with food. She didn't realize that eating this way was causing her to gain weight. She simply ate the junk food her friends were eating. While they appeared content to stop at one, Lauren would go home and make a meal out of it. This only helped to temporarily ease her pain

Lauren, aware that her mother was health-conscious, became creative at finding new places to hide junk food, such as storing her chocolate bars alongside the reclining chair in the living room. Her increasing weight gain each year did not, however, go unnoticed, as her mother would make demeaning comments such as "Lauren, you're gaining so much weight," or "Lauren, you're looking fat." Lauren resented her mother, feeling unsupported and unloved by her. She told me, "I felt that she didn't love me, that she was judging me all the time." Lauren, knowing how her mother felt about ice cream, recalled going straight to the store for a large cone on the heels of a disparaging remark her mother made.

Feeling bad about her increased weight gain, Lauren began holding her chin up in an attempt to make herself look thinner. She was good at convincing others she was overweight through no fault of her own by the controlled way she ate in front of them. In truth, Lauren had become a closet eater who ate alone anytime she got the chance and would often eat from morning until night.

One of Lauren's frequent after-school binges would begin with four chocolate bars, a large bag of potato chips, a quart of ice cream, and a tub of Betty Crocker icing. Dinner would be followed with a large bag of cheezies and a bowl of cereal before going to bed. Hearing this brought back my own past memories, and with them, the fierce determination to teach others how the Method can help free them from this prison.

Realizing now that the root of her overeating was connected to her father, Lauren set to the task of resolving it. She began with a visualization asking him why he had treated her this way. This proved difficult because her father had his guard up and Lauren was unable to get through to him. She remembered that she would need to speak to him past his guard by looking into that quiet, reflective place in his mind. In speaking to her father this way, Lauren began to understand him. She saw how he felt trapped trying to be what his father wanted and how he lost his identity in the pursuit to secure his love and acceptance. In understanding this, Lauren was able to feel compassion for him. In sensing her compassion, her father let his guard down, enabling him to honestly and openly acknowledge what he had done.

Lauren, now able to get through to her father, told him what his abusive behaviour had done to her and how it had affected their relationship. She could feel his remorse and sorrow. This opened her heart, enabling her to forgive him. Lauren then asked her father something she always wanted to know but was too fearful of what she might hear. She asked him how he felt about her, if he loved her. He told her that he loved her very deeply and hated himself for everything he had done. Lauren needed to hear this, as it was crucial to the healing process. Toward the end of the visualization, she gave her father a gift, an opportunity to see the possibilities that life had to offer when he loved and accepted who he was. Lauren felt a release in her chest and a calmness she could not remember feeling before.

It had been months since Lauren last spoke to her father. For reasons she could not explain, Lauren felt compelled to call him. She said, "Dad, I want to ask you a question. Do you miss me?" "Every day," he replied. "I pray every day that you're happy." He told her he was proud of her and of everything she had accomplished and that he loved her. For Lauren and her father, this was the beginning of the healing process.

Not long after this conversation, her father began to attend Al-Anon, a support group for family members of alcoholics. He came to the realization that he wanted to discover his authentic self and purpose in life. Lauren's father has come full circle and now finds fulfillment in giving lectures on anger management.

Lauren has found herself amidst many positive changes. While working on the root of her over-eating, she happened to notice the cravings were gone. Lauren described this as a subtle, yet powerful change, just as I had experienced many years before. She found it astonishing that something so strong, so all encompassing, just stopped. To her, this was nothing short of a miracle.

After the first month, Lauren was elated but skeptical that this would not last. Although she was fearful the cravings would return, they didn't. She could not believe this long nightmare had ended. During the following two months, Lauren noticed a shift, a change in herself. It was a quiet knowledge that the overeating and constant cravings were gone. Once Lauren was able to get to the root of her problem, the overeating stopped. She knew that chapter of her life had come to a close and was now about to embark on a new journey.

Lauren feels stronger, healthier, and more balanced, and, above all, has managed to lose 30 pounds in four months without dieting – and is still losing. She has begun to think of herself as a thin person. In the past, when she ate, regardless of what it was, Lauren would think it was making her gain weight. Now when she eats, she visualizes food nourishing her body, keeping her strong, slender, and healthy.

The most important change, however, is how Lauren feels about herself. She told me, "I always thought I'd like myself once I became skinny, but I realize now that you have to like yourself first." In working through these past issues, Lauren was able to change her beliefs about herself and, in the process, learn the power of forgiveness.

Lauren recently told me she now has the confidence to stand up for herself and speak her mind, especially with her father. She is free from the past and now feels in control of her life and her emotions. Lauren has also been able to let go of the many destructive beliefs about herself. She wrote, "Children are inherently lovable. If my parents couldn't show me that they loved me, it is because they weren't shown love themselves. It had nothing to do with me. I was a bright and happy little girl and I deserve to be happy and healthy. Thank you, Lana, for helping me discover this truth. The child in me is jumping up and down with joy."

10

My Story

We must all be open,
not only to just hearing our inner voice of survival,
but also listening to it.

I woke up to find that nothing had changed. The last thought I had before falling asleep was how amazing it would be to wake up free from the cravings. They say that if you think positive thoughts before you sleep, your mind will continue to focus on them during the night. But lying there on my bed, I could already feel the last vestige of hope slipping away like sand through my fingers. This day would be just like the rest of them. I dragged myself out of bed and into the car, trying to shake off the fogginess in my head. Standing in line at the grocery store, it suddenly occurred to me that I didn't remember getting there. Looking down at the packages of donuts in my hands, I felt increasingly despondent.

I finished the last bit of sugar-laden donut as I sat in the driveway. I felt exhausted. I just wanted to die. I prayed for God to take my life. This was the one time I had felt closer to God than ever before. I could feel his presence. It was as if he were taking care of me, preventing anything from happening. It had also been the one time I felt closest to the other side. I was almost in a dreamlike state, half of me here, the other half there. How the hell, I wondered, did I ever get to this point in my life?

I grew up in a family of seven. Mine was your average typical family of the early 1960's. Back then it was not uncommon to see families with five or six children. This was a time when people didn't seem to worry about whether or not they could afford to have more children, they just did, and mine was no exception. My mother was a stay-at-home mom as were most moms in our neighbourhood. My father was the breadwinner who left early and came home late. We owned our own home on a postage stamp sized lot in suburbia and drove a dark blue, four-door Pontiac sedan.

Living on a tight budget, my mother learned to cut corners wherever possible. It was always the same thing, shepherd's pie, canned soup and vegetables, Swanson's frozen TV dinners, and fruit cocktail (the one that had only two cherries in the can, which everyone fought over.) We drank powdered milk and had the occasional roast chicken and potatoes. Sundays we looked forward to because it meant traditional home-cooked spaghetti with meatballs.

At school, lunch consisted of a peanut butter sandwich, a thermos full of milk, and a piece of fruit. I ate this every day from Grade 6 throughout high school. The tedium of eating the same thing day in and day out left me feeling deprived. It's no small wonder I was always thinking about food, and consequently spent the better part of my senior years drooling over everyone else's lunch. On occasion, my friends would give me a cookie or whatever tidbit they didn't feel like eating, and I would devour it as though it were my last meal. I was convinced they only did this because they felt sorry for me. If my mother had occasionally put cookies or something different to eat in my lunch instead of the same tired thing, then possibly I would not have focused so much on food.

With five kids in our family, sweets never lasted very long. On Sunday we would buy fresh donuts from the bakery on our way home after church; these were devoured in less than five minutes. Unfortunately, we would only get one each. I would dream of the day I could eat as many donuts as I wanted.

Halloween – how we looked forward to it. We would come home after an hour or so of trick-or-treating with bags full of candy. My mother, sitting cross-legged in front of the TV, would have us empty them, leaving us to again take to the streets in our quest for more. After she sifted through everything, keeping only the ones she preferred, would she allow us to have the rest. My father, inherently sensing my mother's lenience with candy, put all our bags in the trunk of his car. He informed us that we could choose only one treat per week, his reason, being the many cavities we were falling victim to, not to mention the escalating dental bills. However, my father's sweet tooth kept him busy, and it wasn't until later that I realized why the pickings were so slim.

With occasional Saturdays came the wonderful aroma of freshly baked butter tarts. We stood by watching, our mouths watering, as our mother counted out 100 tarts cooling on the table. Her tarts melted in your mouth, with just the right amount of crunch. We were allowed to eat as many as we wanted and, believe me, like a pack of hungry wolves, we did. Imagine over the course of a weekend eating 100 butter tarts among the six of us. We gorged ourselves because it was either feast or famine, and if you didn't jump in there and push your way to the front to get your share, then you risked missing out altogether.

Outings would always revolve around food, and it seemed that they were only about food. I remember my mother taking us on a picnic. She packed up a lunch, we walked to the park, ate, and then walked home. There was no hiking, no swimming, or even throwing around a ball. I use to wonder why my mother went through all that trouble, only to turn around and come right back home after eating. To my mind, that's not how I imagined a picnic to be.

Road trips were also quite similar. My mother would pack up the car with licorice, chocolate bars, pop, fruit, and nuts. We had not even driven beyond the city limits and we were already stuffed, everything devoured. I later realized that I was the unknowing recipient of my mother's tumultuous relationship with food.

The age of 7 was a major turning point for me. I experienced a grand mal seizure and was hospitalized for three weeks. I was further warned I would experience migraine headaches upon returning home. That summer was exceptionally hot, as we had not yet enjoyed the benefits of air conditioning. I remember sitting on the kitchen chair in the suffocating heat, holding my head in my hands, rocking back and forth, crying out in pain. I believed, like most children, my mother had the power to make the pain go away. But there was nothing she could do except console me.

The doctors informed my parents that I had some minimal brain damage. At the time, they believed that this damage could affect my intelligence and learning capacity. This belief, however, became an excuse perpetuated by my parents and then me for the many future problems I was to later encounter. Also, at that time, I began taking seizure medication, which acted as a mild sedative. My mother felt that after my seizure, I had gone from an outgoing child to a quiet and solemn child. This further instilled the belief that the seizure had changed me, changed who I was. I eventually came to understand it was the medication that affected my change in personality, but, at the time, the brain damage was perceived to be the sole cause.

During this time, I was experiencing some upsetting problems at school with the other children. It began with a silly schoolyard game of tag where we would scream out, "You've got the cooties!" This was fine and well until the day it was announced that I had the cooties...permanently. From that day on, word spread, and the teasing and cruelty continued through Junior High.

In addition, the school I attended consisted of predominantly caucasian children, where I was the minority. Being of Italian descent with dark skin and dark hair, I then earned a name, an offensive and distasteful word I refer to as the "N" word, often racially associated with people of a darker persuasion. This left me feeling different from the others, centered out, and terribly alone. I felt I was the only one who was made fun of. This name calling and ostracism continued from Grade 2 throughout the beginning of Grade 9, when it abruptly stopped. At that age, it was considered uncool to openly name-call, often resulting in the redirection of the insult back to its rightful owner.

To make matters worse, I felt I was the least liked by the teachers, as they would always sit me in the back corner of the classroom. My last name started with a Z, and I didn't realize until later that back in the 1960's it was common practice to sit children in alphabetical order.

I was a Catholic attending a Protestant school, which was not without its own difficulties. I recall one particular day as my teacher was handing out Bibles to the class, overhearing her remark to her assistant, "She doesn't get a Bible, she's Catholic." Every morning found me watching all my classmates reading from the Bible while I had to stand there feeling increasingly uncomfortable and alienated. I found this to be quite confusing because, as a Catholic, I also read from a Bible. This only further instilled my belief there was something wrong with me, that I was different from the rest.

At the age of 11, my father died. He lost his battle to pancreatic cancer within just four short months. At that point, the accumulation of life's events became too much for me to handle. I had this fear that my life, as I knew it, was coming to an end. I felt alone in a house full of people. I was also feeling unstable and worried that we would have to move to the poor side of town.

My mother had very little control over my siblings, without my father there to set boundaries. I realized I had to be the one to provide stability for them in his place. My mother's way of dealing with her pain was to immerse herself in front of the TV, which, in turn, made me feel I had to hold things together tighter still.

During my father's illness, I was sent to stay with relatives so he could have peace and quiet during the last few weeks of his life. Unaware that my father was dying, I unknowingly developed similar sympathy pains and spent a lot of time agonizing over my own imagined impending death. Shortly after returning home, I overheard my father talking amongst friends about the symptoms of his illness. To my shock and surprise, they were the same symptoms I had been experiencing, but when I said as much, no one responded, no one said anything. I felt alone and had no one to turn to.

My mother, at the young age of 32, found herself a widow with five young children ranging in age from 6 to 11. When she met my father at age 17, he was 20 years her senior and to her represented a father figure. He took care of her; in essence she was like his little girl. Now she was faced with raising us completely on her own.

Because my mother married at such a young age, she felt she had somehow missed her youth and longed to recapture it. As my mother was very beautiful, there was no shortage of men who sought her company. This was a newfound freedom for her, and she spent a great deal of time socializing and dating. Although ultimately no man came before her children, and, to her credit, she wasted no time making this clear to the men she spent time with. She loved each and every one of us very much, and, because of this, we never felt she was acting out of selfishness.

I felt it was my duty to take care of the family after the death of my father because it was what I believed he would have wanted. I have always been mature for my age, and, as the oldest, took it upon myself to act as surrogate mother to my siblings. In some ways I also became a mother to my own mother.

My father never liked having his personal items touched or tampered with, so in my attempt to further honour his memory, I made sure that his things were put away in a safe place. He always liked a clean and tidy home and would become upset if things were disorganized and messy. In order to ensure that everything was as it should be, I would clean the house and do the laundry every day. Many evenings found me up well past ten o'clock organizing last-minute details and setting the breakfast table for the following morning. At lunch, I would run home from school to do the breakfast dishes and tidy up anything else that was out of place. I always felt that my father was watching over me and that he was very proud. This further reinforced the need to continue with this ritual.

Shortly after my father's death, food became my everything. It comforted me and made me feel content. I learned how to bake in order to fulfill my cravings because then I could make what I wanted and eat until I was stuffed. In one afternoon alone, I would bake a couple of dozen cookies or a lemon loaf and eat most of it while watching TV. This became my favourite pastime.

I looked forward to my trips to the bakery. Armed with a bag full of pastries, I would scout the park for a secluded place where I was sure not to be seen. I never considered bringing them home because then I would have to share them with everyone else.

A part of me knew my relationship with food was not normal, yet I just could not stop myself from behaving this way. I sometimes wondered how life would be to think and feel like other kids who could play all day without giving a thought toward food or skip dinner because I was so involved in what I was doing that it wouldn't even occur to me to eat. Needless to say, in time, this behaviour caught up with me, as it did not come without the obvious consequences.

During my mid-to-late teens, I struggled to keep my weight down in order to look and feel attractive. Evenings out with my friends were spent enjoying myself without even so much as a passing thought toward food, until I got home. The first thing I would do is change into my loose-fitting clothes, then sit with my mother in front of the TV, and proceed to eat my way into the early hours of the morning.

I felt as though I were two different people, leading two separate lives. There was the me that wanted to be beautiful, slim, and have it all together. And then there was the other me who was content to spend my time at home eating. To make up for my regression and to absolve myself of this behaviour, I would go on a fast, thinking I could bring myself down to what I thought would be a thinner, more acceptable weight.

This ritual gave me the confidence to feel better about myself and feel more attractive.

The cravings and overeating continued, and with it came the drastic measures I took to stay in control – countless diet pills, laxatives and enemas, not to mention any and all of the latest weekly fad diets readily available. No matter how ridiculous, I tried them all, yet throughout this turmoil I made the decision to go to college at the age of 24. I had a purpose, a direction, and was going to complete my education and finally become something. Then things started to change. The stress was mounting, my relationship ended abruptly, and I was feeling threatened by someone from my past. My life had begun to unravel.

I recall more than once during my classes suddenly becoming overwhelmed with strong cravings. It became increasingly difficult to remain focused. Thoughts of food began to consume me, affecting my concentration. I immediately left the class to satisfy my craving. I ate and ate until I felt a sense of relief wash over me. My body relaxed like a drug addict who just got a fix. Within minutes, a feeling of remorse welled up inside. I justified this by telling myself it was okay; it was just one little setback. However, I knew the bakery on the drive home would prove to be the ultimate test, and the many afternoons that followed found me sitting in the parking lot where I proceeded to finish an entire log cake before going home. The more I ate, the more I craved. I just could not stop myself. I felt like a complete failure. I was living in my own private hell, feeling that no one could possibly understand or help me.

Eventually, driving by the bakery became so difficult that I found myself looking for an alternate route to avoid the temptation. Like all other previous attempts, this proved unsuccessful. My classmates said nothing. They didn't have to. I could feel them watching me as I continued to expand. And expand I did at a rapid pace. In just one month I gained 25 pounds and I could see this was only just the beginning.

I remember standing in front of my closet in despair, separating the fat clothes from the thin and feeling if I didn't hurry up and find something that didn't make me look fat, I would never get out of the house. I knew if I didn't leave then, I never would. Quitting school just wasn't an option because it was all I had left to hold onto in the hope of making a success of myself.

Now single, I felt there was no reason for me to stay thin. I later realized I could not be thin for someone else because as soon as that person was out of my life, the weight would be regained through my own destructive behaviour. I had to do it for me, not for anyone else. I had to love myself before anyone else could.

I was wearing down and I knew I was nearing the end of my rope. As a result of the breakup, the rapidly progressing weight gain, and weariness of years spent struggling with this, I had become very depressed. I felt trapped. There was no way out. Things escalated. Physically ill and emotionally drained, I would fall, exhausted, into an uneasy, restless sleep, only to awake and face yet another day of suffering. I felt completely defeated and could not go through this again, only to fail miserably.

My mother, able to see just how much I was suffering, called someone she believed could help. I felt comfortable with this person and over time came to regard him as not only a close friend but also a trusted mentor. Our relationship grew as a result of a deep respect for one another. He was able to help me immensely, introducing me to the art of visualization. This, for me, proved to be the first step in the right direction.

I thought back to when at age 14, a friend, who possessed amazing insight, always maintained that my problem with food was connected to my father. At the time, I was unable to see this connection and reacted defensively because I idolized my father and was not open to having someone defame his character. However, after 13 years and many failed attempts to lose weight, I was willing to entertain the possibility she may be right, and I was ready to try anything that would help me feel normal again.

148

So began my vigilant pursuit to work on issues involving my father by using visualization a few minutes each night. Throughout this time I remained hopeful and relieved that I was finally making progress toward healing myself. My life had begun to turn around; it felt as though a gray cloud had lifted. I was happy. Life was good.

With diligence, it did not take long before my struggle with food came to an end. It was an amazing feeling and an amazing process. There are no words to describe the freedom I felt with food no longer nagging at me day and night. I stopped planning and revolving my life around food. I stopped thinking about it, obsessing about it, and agonizing over it. Food was no longer my focus or the centre of my life.

Looking back on this troubling time, it still amazes me that I was able to crawl out from under this mess. It did not, however, come without great personal cost, which took a tremendous toll on me both mentally and physically. Hitting this low point enabled me to realize that no diet in the world was the answer, and the only solution would be to look for the reasons why I was behaving this way. Writing this book has not only been therapeutic but also a meaningful way for me to reach out and help others.

When I overcame my struggle, 25 years ago, it was essentially a hit and miss process. I experimented with different ideas, hoping something would work. This eventually led me to what is now known as the "Method." I lost 35 pounds and have effortlessly kept it off for over 25 years.

Today I am still able to eat what I want without having to worry about gaining weight and losing control. Food no longer has the same hold over me it once had. Looking at myself today, I cannot believe that person was me. That person no longer exists. It is all now a distant memory – a lifetime ago.

11

Okay, Now That I'm Thin... What Next?

....

Putting the Method to Work When Life's Problems Get in the Way

> *When we get to wherever it is we want to go*
> *and put all our energy into getting there,*
> *we stand unsure of ourselves as to what to do next.*
> *It is in just being there that we need to celebrate*
> *our victories, ourselves, and our lives to the fullest.*

When I overcame my struggle with food, I realized my eating problem was only a manifestation of the larger issues that lay below. With that in mind, I knew the Method would be beneficial for the many other issues that we encounter apart from overeating. I decided then to put it to the test, and, with much success, it delivered time and time again.

Lara

Often, as children, we are made to feel small even though we don't feel this way. Unfortunately, the severity of this treatment can have a lasting and debilitating effect.

Lara, 26, asked for help with a fear she was encountering that seemingly began to take over and cripple her life. Lara finds herself afraid to ask for help. She is afraid to call about a problem or inquiry, afraid to ask for assistance if she can't find what she is looking for, even afraid to call a restaurant to make a reservation. When Lara does ask for help, people respond rudely, leaving her feeling helpless and defeated.

This proved to be a constant struggle for Lara, as she felt she was not on an equal playing field. As a result, when Lara was in this situation, she would become submissive, unable to stand up for herself. Lara reached a point where she began to worry about how people would treat her in most situations. Even buying a pack of gum or ordering a pizza proved difficult without suffering from the accompanying feelings of anxiety. This had become an unbearable and consistent pattern in Lara's life.

Using the Method to find the root of her problem, I asked Lara to think back to the earliest incident, one that reminded her of this issue. She remembered one that occurred when she was 10 years old. It is important to note that, for Lara, just having a recollection of this memory enabled her to feel a release of some of the pressure and anxiety. This is not uncommon for some people to experience when connecting it back to the root of their problem.

At the age of 10, Lara had come up with the very creative idea of having a Piñata at her aunt's shower. In the midst of her excitement, she began to call the stores to locate one. Lara's request was met with a very condescending and unhelpful response. She recalled, as she spoke with the salesperson, that she could feel herself shrinking. Defeated, Lara could not find the courage to ask for further help. Because of how this left her feeling, she allowed her creative idea to fall through.

With this visualization, Lara was able to realize that this woman, whose primary job was to assist customers with respect regardless of their age, was clearly out of line. Had Lara or her parents lodged a complaint about this salesperson, she would have, in all probability, been held accountable for her behaviour. This fact in and of itself gave Lara back her power, which was something she desperately needed. She realized that she was and is worthy of others' help and assistance, which helped change her core belief.

Lara also realized that this was only one incident in her life and it should not dictate what happens with every future incident. She was able to see how foolish and unnecessary her fear had been all along.

She found herself saying, "Oh, is that all it was? Is that where this came from? I can't believe I reacted so fearfully over something like that all these years." With this realization, something in Lara changed; she felt a release and a feeling of lightness that often accompanies resolving issues.

Lara, now more confident and self-assured, has found that when she asks for help, people are quite accommodating and most often go out of their way for her. The interesting part is that this is neither forced nor practiced but comes naturally and effortlessly to her.

My Employer

There are times in life when we come to a crossroad and need to make a decision. One way is the easy road of escape, whereas the other, we know, is the difficult one. But we realize, in the end, the easier road is not always the best.

A number of years ago, I had an employer who became quite irate with me for work he felt was incomplete. It was a procedure I was not aware that needed to be implemented. He not only stated that it was my responsibility to have known this but also expected it, despite the fact I had not received prior training. Although this may have been an error on my part, I felt the severity of his anger to be unwarranted. Simply pointing out what was required would have been more appropriate.

This incident really bothered and upset me. I wanted to quit. I asked myself if I should find another job or stay and work it out. After struggling for some time over this, I realized the only answer was to resolve the issue, not run from it. If I were to run from this without working it out, then I would, without a doubt, find myself again in a similar situation.

Using the Method to find the root of my problem, I remembered the earliest incident that reminded me of this one. I recalled my father becoming angry with me for things I didn't realize I had done. Even though I was diligent at whatever I attempted, regardless of how hard I worked or tried, it felt as though it was never enough. I realized that the root of this issue was with my father, not my employer, and it was there that I began to work it out.

When my father was disapproving and angry with me, I perceived that the world was angry with me. As a result, I came to believe I was not worthy, that I was this bad little girl who didn't deserve to have good things happen to her. I could see this belief was present whenever others expressed their disapproval. I realize now, reflecting on this belief, how ridiculous it was for me to feel this way. The world was not mad at me, and I was deserving of good things.

This is often how experiences can be erroneously perceived through a child's eyes and then carried into adulthood, resulting in the "hang-ups" and "excessive baggage" we so often hear about. I was a good child, and any wrongdoing I may have done, I knew, was not intentional.

These facts, brought to light, were crucial for me to understand in order to begin the healing process. I

157

came to realize, looking now through adult eyes, that my father, at that time in his life, had many worries and was quite possibly at the beginning stages of the disease that would ultimately claim his life. He was also a product of his own childhood, coming from a time when "children were to be seen and not heard" and therefore would have felt that his response or lack thereof was an appropriate way to behave toward his child.

Using the Method, I visualized my father at the time of the incident, telling him how I felt about what he had done and how unfairly he had treated me. He stood listening as I spoke. I was able to release the hurt I had been holding on to, yet I was still feeling upset. It was the realization that he had wasted so much of the precious time we had together reprimanding and disciplining me that it left little time for the things that mattered. I could see that my father agreed the years were squandered on harsh discipline, not love. I then dissolved into tears, feeling a release in my chest and a release of the anger I had harboured toward him.

This visualization proved to be a crucial turning point for me. To determine its success, I visualized my boss. I could see his expression soften as he spoke from his heart saying he did not want me to leave and valued me not only as the likable, caring person he believed me to be, but also the consummate professional he knew I was.

The results of the Method were twofold. Not only did it change the relationship between my boss and I for the better but also I was able to resolve this repetitive, longstanding issue from my childhood.

Samantha

We go through life looking at our problems as a thorn in our side, wondering why things always happen to us. Close relationships can become a challenge, as they are often not as harmonious as we would wish them to be. And due to the nature of our circumstances, they are not ones that can easily be walked away from. We need to look at them as a message that will lead us to the root of our problem because it is there that we will find the answers. This is the place where we begin.

Samantha came to me upset about the altercations she was regularly having with her 8 year old daughter. She realized these fights centred around her daughter's need to exercise control over most situations. Whenever Sam had an argument with her, she found herself experiencing anger to the point of shaking. Feeling victimized, she kept asking, "Why is this happening to me? What did I do to deserve this?" Aware that she was blowing it out of proportion, Sam could not understand why she felt so emotional over this and had no idea how to begin dealing with these feelings.

Taking a look at the problem, I was able to show Sam that the constant battles she and her daughter were having indicated a clear message that pointed to a past unresolved conflict she had with her own mother. Sam recalled that the power struggle between her and her mother was very similar to the one she was experiencing with her daughter.

The Method gave Samantha the ability and know-how to work on it, and as she did, she noticed that the feelings of anger and the irrational emotions she was experiencing stopped. She no longer looked at herself as the victim or blamed her daughter for the arguments and altercations they were having. As a result, she was able to take responsibility for this problem and overcome it.

Yvette

To discipline means to teach. And we learn through these teachings at an early age the basics of right and wrong, what is acceptable and what is not, and that our actions have consequences which often result in punishment. But sometimes we interpret these punishments in ways that impede our emotional growth in adulthood. These occurrences need to be resolved in order to move forward.

One woman credits the Method for helping her to overcome what she had always felt to be one of her most troublesome problems. Had it not been for the Method, she would not have experienced the major breakthrough that resulted in transforming her life.

Yvette recently failed her state-licensing exam. She couldn't understand it because she had studied hard and believed herself to be well prepared. Yvette felt her world had fallen apart. She was unable to see that this was actually a blessing in disguise.

Perplexed as to how this could have happened, Yvette turned to the Method. She realized that she had felt dominated and at the mercy of the licensing board. Yvette also realized that she had experienced the same feeling with her employers, who were forever attempting to exercise control over her. To Yvette's surprise, this had become a pattern in many aspects of her life.

Yvette asked herself what this reminded her of. Her earliest memory was that of her mother sending her to her room as punishment whenever she felt a lesson needed to be learned. The many hours spent in solitude allowed a deep resentment to grow. She recalled feeling overpowered and dominated by her mother.

Yvette knew she needed to resolve this pattern of domination or it would continue to suppress her permanently. As she visualized this scene, Yvette spoke to her mother, explaining how her discipline and control had had such a negative and lasting impact on her and how it, as a result, prevented her from advancing in her career and her life. Yvette spoke about how her inner strength had been suppressed and that this strength was to be used in a positive way in order to make a difference.

This visualization for Yvette was a step forward. She felt a powerful release and experienced a renewed feeling of confidence. The same day, Yvette quit her job. She felt calm and assertive, coming from a place of strength. Her employers expressed sadness and were surprised with her decision.

Not long afterward, Yvette passed her licensing exam with flying colours and has now started her own business, which promises to be a success. Overcoming this problem has not only changed the course of Yvette's life but has also given her the fortitude and vision to move forward and make a difference.

As we move through life, we discover we are never immune to the challenges we face. As these diverse narratives illustrate, the Method has the ability to absolve us from the many problems that hold us back.

The above examples describe those who have reaped the benefits of the Method. They were not only able to understand their behaviours and reactions to these situations but they also learned how to put an end to the repetitive patterns and fears that were crippling their lives. If used frankly and honestly, the Method will enable us to face these problems with newfound knowledge and the courage to resolve them.

164

It is my sincere hope that you accomplish everything you set out to achieve. I know the Method has fulfilled this for me – even beyond my own expectations.

ABOUT THE AUTHORS

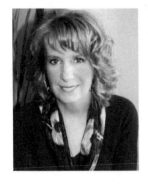

Kim Cutulle is and has always been a keen observer of the human condition. Her insights into life's triumphs, failures, and ironies make her an honest witness to her times. While getting her point across with an economy of words, it is in the roles of sounding board, devil's advocate, soul mate, and muse that Kim helps Lana bring her story to these pages. Kim lives with her husband, children, and assorted pets in a rural community near Grimsby, Ontario, Canada.

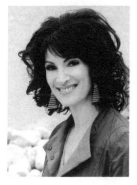

Lana Zincone struggled with her weight for many years, and in her search for the underlying reasons why she could not stop overeating, developed a method enabling her to find the root of her problem. Lana lost 35 pounds and has effortlessly kept it off for over 25 years.

The inspiration for writing this book was born as the result not only of Lana's experience and that of others, but also of the many inquiries of how she achieved permanent success with her Method. It is her hope that it will strike a resonating chord, inspire her readers and prove just how strong and resilient they can be when challenged with life's obstacles and emerge triumphant. Lana lives with her husband and children in Waterloo, Ontario, Canada.

Printed in Poland
by Amazon Fulfillment
Poland Sp. z o.o., Wrocław

25488477R00107